MEDICINE, TRADITION, AND DEVELOPMENT IN KENYA AND TANZANIA, 1920–1970

MEDICINE, TRADITION, AND DEVELOPMENT IN KENYA AND TANZANIA, 1920–1970

by

Ann Beck

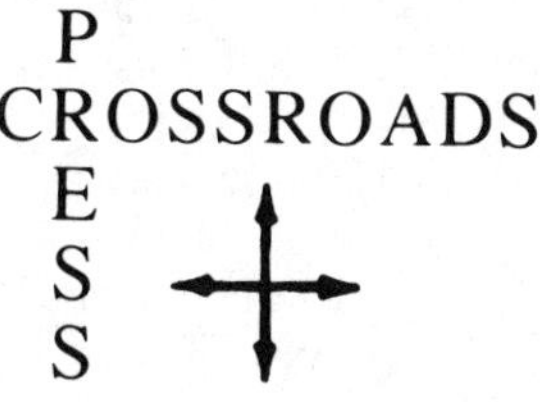

International Standard Book Number 0-918456-44-4

Crossroads Press
Epstein Building, Brandeis University
Waltham, Massachusetts 02254

(Crossroads Press is a subsidiary
of the African Studies Association)

Printed in the United States of America

CONTENTS

ACKNOWLEDGEMENTS

This study was in part supported by Grant No. 2 ROI-LMO 803-4 from the National Library of Medicine, whose help I deeply appreciate. I am grateful to the University of Hartford for its assistance in the preparation of the manuscript for publication. Professors Bill Brayfield and David Courtwright of the History Department of the University of Hartford gave me the benefit of their critique. Professor Brayfield read the first four chapters of the manuscript. His penetrating critique made me rethink my assumptions and conclusions. Dr. David Courtwright read the entire manuscript. His editorial comments and suggestions were very valuable to me. Professor Cranford Pratt of the University of Toronto, though not in agreement with my historical approach to the problems of political economy in Tanzania, made me aware of my imperfections. I also appreciated Professor Mburu's comments, who–as Senior Lecturer in Community Health at the University of Nairobi–gave me a different perspective for my evaluation of medicine and development in East Africa.

This book could not have been written without the personal contact and the individual discussions with a number of professors and postgraduates at the Universities of Dar es Salaam and Nairobi and with the many officials who gave me freely of their time to answer my questions. Most of all, however, the reality of Africa itself helped me to test theories and models in the light of the everyday normal life of Kenya and Tanzania.

PREFACE

The transformation of societies through industrialization, technology, and science in the nineteenth century led to the increasingly widespread acceptance of cultural progress and socio-economic development as desirable goals for modern man, whose rising standard of living would be guaranteed for the continued growth of production and mass consumption. Economists and social planners identified development with the continuing capacity of public and private enterprise to satisfy the needs of a modern mass society, a society which assumed the beneficence of this process and the generalization of the progress thus achieved.

In the colonial societies of the industrialized imperialist nations, however, different trends became apparent. Developmental planning accepted in the western world was not introduced in the African economies until 1929, and such planning did not affect the laborers and peasants there until after World War II. Even then, such planning was limited to projects of general improvement in selected areas such as transportation, administrative services, agricultural production for export, and the cultivation of basic food for rural populations. One reason for this long delay was that Colonial development schemes came at an unfortunate time: the onset of the world depression in 1929. Further delay was caused by the years of economic stagnation before World War II.[1]

Many theories of development have been presented during the last decades in an attempt to induce or to evaluate economic growth in its relation to demographic changes and human aspirations. One variant of such theories, the theories of "underdevelopment," tend to stress the disadvantages which the former colonies had to face after independence, as well as the special local conditions not conducive to western patterns of growth.

It is not the intention of this book to add to the ideological controversaries and the economic analyses of the vast and still growing literature on underdevelopment. However, both Kenya and Tanzania opted for economic planning as soon as they became independent states after 1960, and thus faced from the beginning the issue of development; they were forced to choose between radical socio-economic change or more conservative programmatic aspirations. For this reason, some of the theories of development applicable to East Africa will be referred to briefly.

The major concern of this study is to portray the experiments, programs, and policies attempted during the transition to independence and in the years thereafter, especially those involving public health, modern medicine, and traditional medical practices in Kenya and Tanzania.[2] This should illustrate many aspects of their history during the last forty years. The study will also explore the process of devolution from colonial administration to the establishment of a new political basis capable of transforming nineteenth-century agricultural economies into the technologically sophisticated world of the mid-twentieth century. Forced to respond to world-wide trends while struggling to maintain their special character as predominantly rural societies, the goals and criteria of development of the western world had to be modified or changed if they were to serve as guides in the less-developed countries of East Africa.

1

DEVELOPMENT IN COLONIAL EAST AFRICA AFTER 1920: THE FORMULATION OF GOALS

Long before the first Development Act was introduced in 1929, colonial policy statements referred to the need for development, though they did not define it strictly. Development might refer to a vaguely conceived "advancement of civilization" in East Africa, the improvement of skills among African peasants to make their labor output more productive, the improvement of roads and transport to stimulate commerce, the raising of overall productivity in the "interest of humanity" and the expansion of African agriculture for the sake of Africans and Europeans alike.[1] Most of the official and unofficial references were couched in general terms and did not lend themselves to practical application until 1923, when a bill was proposed giving the Secretary of State power to subsidize Imperial development schemes.[2] During this period plans for development were not based on economic or social theories and did not immediately affect colonial policy after World War I.

Also during this period the term "underdevelopment" was not used in describing the economics of Kenya and Tanzania. Contemporary liberal opinion criticized government for its failure to advance African civilization because it overlooked the importance of extended contacts between western civilization and that of the Africans, thereby not giving them a chance to gain from European initiative and enterprise.[3] This failure, they believed, was due to Britain's post-war stagnation which forced her to concentrate her energies on new economic and social policies at home.

What could be done for East Africa after World War I? Two sets of objectives were proposed. One was the upgrading of the European economic sector in Africa; the other was the social improvement of the African population. To help Europeans in Africa and to relieve British unemployment at home, it was proposed to raise agricultural production and to increase empire trade. England accepted her obligation to the African people, the majority of whom were peasants, thought to be not yet able to help themselves to improve their economic and social condition. From the start of planning, therefore, the policy for African development was circumscribed by government interpretations of the African capabilities. The two sets of objectives were pursued by colonial authorities with varying degrees of urgency. In a memorandum on native policy in 1930, which explained Britain's specific obligations toward African peasants, it was argued that although the colonial government had introduced a modern administration, it had not taught the natives how to use it. Government, therefore, wished to assume responsibility in this respect, hoping thereby "to promote the development of the resources of [the] territory and prosperity of its inhabitants, including the immigrant communities within it." In particular, the prosperity of the Africans required a "progressive raising of the economic standard of life." The material surroundings in which Africans lived, therefore, and provisions for medical facilities, hospitals and dispensaries should be regarded as of equal importance with the supply of teachers and schools. The colonial government should also aim to train natives to take care of their own services through local councils.[4]

The Development Act of 1929 went through a long process of maturation before it finally became law. But even then it did not perceptibly change colonial policy or colonial production. The small steps taken towards development before 1929 are characteristic of the final result. They reflect cautious pragmatism and the conviction that the economy must be controlled by Europeans until such a time as the African reaches a stage in which he can plan his own advancement and select for himself the quality of life.

The economic crisis in Britain from 1919 to 1922 compelled the postwar government to adopt drastic steps to fight against inflation and unemployment in order to avoid the lingering threat of the radicalization of the masses. Plans for development in eastern Africa were, therefore, subordinated to Britain's all-out effort to overcome serious problems facing home society and politics. The story of this early stage of East African development has been told in detail by E. A. Brett.[5] He listed a series of steps which complemented each other. First among them was the decision by Lloyd George's Cabinet in 1921 to increase the demand for British goods. It is here that a colonial public works program leading to large orders in Britain would give a substantial boost to the British export industry. After the connection between British trade and colonial public works programs had been established, a further step followed logically. Imperial guarantees for interest-free loans were proposed in order to finance colonial road building, construction of railways and scientific research. By 1929, Brett concluded, a new attitude toward financing colonial development projects had emerged, in spite of the world-wide depression which forced Britain to reduce colonial budgets.[6]

The act of 1929 bears the imprint of those who had participated in framing it during one stage or another of its conception between 1920 and 1929. Instructions dispatched by the Secretary of State to administrators of the non-selfgoverning colonies in August 1929 listed some of the legitimate purposes of grants and loans under the Colonial Development Act. Among them were "Aiding and developing agriculture and industry in colonies . . . thereby promoting commerce with or industry in United Kingdom." To achieve this purpose, scientific research, instruction and experimentation were to be encouraged and grants or loans to non-self-governing colonies not to exceed £1 million were authorized by the Treasury.[7] Like all future advisories dispatched by the Colonial Office, the circulars indicate that development programs must be sound, though not necessarily remunerative at once. This was important because it encouraged administrators to consider long-range programs with a potential for growth, programs helping agricultural production in remote areas, intercolonial communication links like the Zambezi river bridge, and the development of mineral resources and water supplies.

The circulars of 1929 also sound a warning to would-be developers that colonial economic development must promote commerce and industry in England and thereby reduce unemployment.[8] Even though Brett is on firm ground in interpreting the 1929 Development Act within the context of Britain's major unemployment and manufacturing crises of the 1920s, one must not forget that, in the 1930s, the concept of development had shifted toward the inclusion of the African factor in colonial society, a factor not considered before 1920. Brett's emphasis on the accelerated pace of economic planning at a time of inflation, depression and restlessness among the postwar generation in metropolitan Britain reflects the conflicting trends of a country which was declining as a world power and, at the same time, holding on tightly to her colonial empire to which concessions had to be made.[9]

Between 1929 and 1940, the Development Act did not live up to expectations. During the depression years, development planning, though much talked about, was not given priority. The Act provided funds for loans and cash grants, but until the middle of the 1930s, fear of a repeat of another depression, rather than confidence in the future, ruled. The Colonial Office dared not risk new enterprises without a reservoir of an accumulated surplus in the colonial territories. Such thinking is the opposite of development philosophy, which sets its hopes for the future on innovative policies financed by funds voted annually by Parliament and thereby not depending on colonial treasuries. Even though the final report of the Colonial Development Advisory Committee in 1940 said that the dual purpose of the Act, the development of the colonies and the promotion of trade, had been ever present in their minds, the advancement of the colonial people had not been noticeably furthered. This is true, notwithstanding a statement by Lloyd George's Cabinet in 1923 that "while measures of relief and extensions of uncovenanted benefits are being proposed as palliatives in the present crisis, the main policy of Government lies in the direction of development of trade and industry in all their branches, and more particularly of Empire Development and Empire Settlement."[10]

What were the shortcomings of the Act and what was its interpretation by administrators? The concept of development, if not clearly defined, had its built-in contradictions, of which its architects were aware. Just reading the reports of the Colonial Development Advisory Committee in the 1930s and noting their labored attempts to devise a formula for cultural and economic improvement of the African,[11] one sees how frustrated the members of the various committees must have been. The Act of 1929, though saying clearly that development in Africa was in the British interest, also said that its purpose must go far beyond it. East and Central Africa as a whole, the Hilton Young Report said in 1929, had enormous agricultural possibilities, but the variety of its conditions and its proper development required continuous study of all factors and the adaptation of methods to varying conditions.[12] What could the practical planner do with these general and vague assertations? Were they merely meant to procrastinate? I believe that there was a genuine uneasiness about the unknown factors and their impact on development, such factors as, for instance, the inability to foretell to what level and how fast the African could be raised, assuming modern British standards as the measure for African progress. And always, of course, the warning was sounded that "progress must inevitably be slow and a matter of the cumulative reinforcement of civilizing influences," which would raise the economic level to a minimum starting point, as Lord Moyne said in relation to Kenya in 1932.[13]

Development planners seem to have been further confused when they tried to define what they wanted to develop. This was important because it determined how funds were to be divided between capital projects and administrative and functional services, such as roads, bridges, hospitals, schools. Further, the question arose how a colony, unable to provide for its basic ongoing routine services, would make use of development funds for innovative improvements. What criteria, other than the placing of substantial orders in the United Kingdom, should be applied? The Committee did not feel bound solely by considerations of profits for the consumer and businessman in England and contemplated development as a long-range policy which might include the agricultural development in native reserves and ecological surveys in eastern Africa to plan for better crops in the future.[14] In this context, public health, scientific research, and education entered the field, although they were only slowly incorporated into the proposed schemes. Over a ten-year period, however, from 1929 to 1939, projects for the improvement of public health were assigned 13 percent of assistance recommended, or £1,071,224 and in 1939, the last year of the 1929 Development Act, the contribution to public health projects reached 40 percent of the total, or £385,096. Seven percent of the total approved for the ten-year period to 1939 was granted for scientific research, a new trend.[15]

Money issued by the Treasury for the total period (as distinguished from funds allocated for spending) in each budget year was only £5,845,000. As Brett noted, only once did spending reach 75 percent of allocations. The Fund's impact on development did not live up to expectations except in those colonies whose administrators were enterprising enough to exploit the funds for special projects. An example is Tanganyika Territory, a country that had been badly hurt by the depression.[16] Another factor in Tanganyika may also have been its mandatory status which obligated Britain to report on the Territory to the League of Nations.

The task of selecting promising schemes for grants was further complicated by the need simultaneously to stimulate colonial productivity and to produce the proper infrastructure for economic growth: the roads, harbors, and mines. Among the schemes considered by the Advisory Committee during the ten-year tenure of the Act of 1929 were such projects as the elimination of unhygienic facilities associated with housing in wooden huts and their replacement with well-planned concrete houses.[17] At the outbreak of World War II, government separated those proposals which it considered essential for survival during the war from others which, though desirable, had to be temporarily shelved during the national emergency. Nevertheless, the surprising decision was made before the expiration of the Development Act to maintain colonial development on a more comprehensive format than before, and include projects of improvement on a long-range basis.

The new Act of 1940, to last only five years, was the beginning of an extended scheme of development legislation. The Act increased annual spending to £5 million to guarantee more comprehensive projects. The name was changed to the Colonial Development *and* Welfare Act to indicate the new special emphasis to be given social improvement, for it had been found that emphasis on schemes of a capital nature gave too much priority to material development.[18]

Despite the special social emphasis, however, this wartime Act did not have a chance to develop its full potential, and legislation was updated again in 1945. This time the Act did two things: it increased the maximum annual spending from £5 million to £10 million, and it extended the term of operation to ten years. This was to enable colonial government to draft long-range development projects for material as well as for social improvement.[19] On the surface, the difference between the 1940 legislation and that of 1945 does not appear so great; but the search for broader objectives of development indicates uncertainty among the planners on how to effect social change, even in an extended period. And as a Parliamentary Command Paper said in 1940, "the existence of the Fund has not involved any departure from the old principle that a colony should have only those services which it can afford to maintain out of its own resources."[20] Unfortunately, at this stage of colonial government, the revamping of the African rural society could not be done.

In his dispatch to colonial governors in November 1945, the Colonial Secretary hailed the latest development legislation as the beginning of a new chapter in colonial development planning. Was it a new beginning and were its intentions directed toward Africans as much as toward the business community in Africa and England? Did the new legislation inaugurate a new era of agricultural productivity, did it introduce changes in techniques, better education, better medical care and extended control of tropical diseases? In the extended debates on the Development Acts between 1923 and 1945, these questions were raised. The significance of the Acts of 1929, 1940 and 1945 lies less in the appropriation of funds and the improvments that were begun rather than in the mere fact that the colonial development planning had become an item on the colonial agenda.

2

MEDICINE AND DEVELOPMENT PLANNING: THE COLONIAL PERIOD

The success and failure of colonial development plans, widely discussed by scholars in recent years, leave the historian puzzled and intrigued. Why did the transition from colonial status to independence lead to a counterproductive start? The new social structures of the former colonies, burdened with a heritage of scarcity and confounded by a pervasive lack of skills, have been examined in the manner of dead bodies in an anatomical laboratory. Their remains revealed to the scrutinizing scientist the marks of stunted growth and crippling defects. Certainly these post-mortem analyses have been instrumental in suggesting remedies for the future.[1]

Something is missing in this literature, however. The analyses do not fully reflect the reality of the years after 1920, a very important period during which the concept of development became for the first time an issue in East Africa. It was, however, an issue riddled with contradictory and overlapping impulses, impulses which betrayed a narrowness of judgment on the part of some officials and a full awareness of the needs of Africans by others.

Four major aspects of the transition era will be discussed in this and the following chapters, including the transition from speculation on development to concrete projects of development, the changes in direction in medical policy, the increasing concern with conditions in rural areas and plans for the improvement of native agriculture as a means of dealing with demographic problems. Throughout the colonial period, while plans for their future were formulated, Africans remained the passive objects of decisive considerations. This is true in spite of the fact that the plans were designed to prepare the indigenous population ultimately for a new role in the shaping of their own lives in a post-colonial society.

At the start of planning for colonial development in the 1920s, social and economic uncertainty preoccupied the attention of policy makers at Westminster, at the Colonial Office in London, and in the administrators' offices in Africa.[2] The Development Act of 1929 passed through several periods of implementation, periods which did not solely depend on economic problems but also on measures of constitutional and political reorganization contemplated for East Africa at the same time. One learns as much about development policy from reports on specific East African problems as from accounts of the Development Advisory Committee itself.

One of the special projects during the latter part of the 1920s was a proposal for an administrative unification of Kenya, Tanganyika, and Uganda, also called "Closer Union." In the debates on this issue by government missions in East Africa and by members of Parliament in London, development was often introduced as a side issue. It was argued, for instance, that native populations would have to play a major role in any consideration of Closer Union, particularly in relation to the key question of how to raise agricultural productivity in the native sector. It was also admitted that specific directions of development were not clearly defined in official reports. The doctrine of "dual policy," to which Britain was officially committed since 1923, anticipated parallel though equal economic development in the African and European sectors. A caveat was added, however, that it would be difficult to appropriate labor for projects to promote economic growth without damage to total productivity if African development was pushed too fast.[3] Since the Closer Union movement had political as well as economic objectives, it did not necessarily share the approaches to development worked up by the Development Advisory Committee. Interested in the total agricultural output of a unified region, the African contribution would have to play a larger role; and in this context, the question was raised how the African peasant could be trained for a higher level of productivity and how fast he could be accommodated to a more rigid discipline of modern western civilization. The Closer Union people identified development with progress in a European sense, and education, hardly begun, was the prerequisite in their opinion. Dual policy, defined by its supporters as "complimentary development of native and non-native communities," forced the discussion into such areas as cultural characteristics, innate abilities, climate, soil, and labor.[4]

These considerations were different from those of the Development Advisory Committee during its deliberations between 1930 and 1940. The Committee's task was on a much narrower scale: to dispose judiciously of appropriations on an accelerated schedule, selecting projects likely to produce "visible" results in a short time. The conflicts of many diversified interest groups during the debates of development policy in 1930 made the selection of such projects a difficult one. The slow beginning, however, was not necessarily symptomatic of what could be done later. Kenya settlers, for instance, protested the implications of Closer Union. They feared a loss of political power and a threat to their political control of the colony. The Indians in Tanganyika were absolutely opposed to the economic consequences of Closer Union which might deprive them of the monopoly of local trade. And an African chief in the Kilimanjaro area opposed it because he feared that native policy in Tanganyika would be adjusted to a settler-dominated native policy in Kenya. Even the coordination of essential economic services like roads, railways, and postal services was opposed by many.[5]

Aware of the conflicting currents in 1930 and anticipating delays in the process of selecting projects, Secretary of State Lord Passfield recommended a concentration on development schemes which would not require lengthy passage through committees in order to be approved by the Treasury. More controversial subjects like public health, though a foundation for any development scheme, were therefore not among the first selections.

The effectiveness of the first Development Act was impaired by the traumatic impact of the world-wide depression on the thinking of policy makers and colonial administrators.[6] It created attitudes of extreme caution and an unwillingness to invest in capital projects like bridge construction, railway building, and the expansion of the colonial productive capacity because they might produce budgetary deficits. Britain was unwilling to assume a continuing responsibility for subsidies to be paid out of the Imperial Treasury. The old principle that a colony must aim at solvency was still maintained, regardless of whether it was strong enough to be able to afford it or too weak to help itself. Brett maintained that when conditions improved after 1934, the crisis attitudes of administrators and planners remained. When, however, the first Development Act of 1929 was replaced by the Colonial Development and Welfare Acts of 1940 and 1945, the change in the title emphasized a change in thinking. Development and welfare funds were to be earmarked in the future for the development of colonial productive resources as well as the improvement of human wellbeing.[7]

In the area of health, the new approach to welfare spending should have affected public health planning beyond the absolutely bare minimum. Even in this critical sector of society, however, progress was slow. A new structure for a rural health system covering the entire colony of Tanganyika was discussed for over twenty years without producing action. Typical of the conflicting attitudes was the protracted debate on the establishment of a medical training school for African medical assistants. A generous offer of £20,000 as a direct loan was suggested through the Development Committee in 1930 and sanctioned by the Secretary of State. The money was to be used for a School of Medicine in Dar es Salaam.[8] After receipt of the offer, plans were drawn up immediately by the Medical Department in Tanganyika and presented to the Development Committee in 1931. Three months later, the government retrenchment committee recommended not to start the work. Undismayed, the Director of Medical Services presented a further detailed plan for the training of Africans, just one month after the retrenchment notice, which shows what importance he attached to the training school. He gave detailed justification and defined the three categories of African medical personnel which the system needed if it was to serve large numbers: orderlies, dispensers, and sanitary inspectors. He also specified a site for the school and gave assurances that the Development Committee loan of £20,000 was not needed any more. The Secretary of State approved "with reluctance" the postponement of the project even after the Medical Director had made it abundantly clear that medical services in rural areas were the prerequisite for development. Without African paramedical help, the services could not be maintained.[9]

The project remained dormant for five more years and was revived by Dr. Scott, Medical Director in Tanzania in 1936. He listed the precise numbers of trainees that ought to be recruited. His modest proposal was put on the back burner once more because the Director of Education "could see no immediate possibility of finding the number required [for training]." The total number of trainees was set at forty, and these could not be found in Tanganyika in 1936 because the curriculum in the the two junior secondary schools in Dar es Salaam and Tanga did not yet have the tenth standard,[10] considered the minimal requirement for trainees.

In 1939, when the Second Colonial Development Act was about to start, the medical school project was revived again. By now the number of trainees requested was revised upward because female nurses for child and maternity welfare were also included. An African Medical School, it was said, was needed for moral and medical reasons because it was the duty of government "to further the moral and material welfare of the people," a majority of whom lived in areas not covered by European medicine.[11]

In further correspondence with the Development Committee,[12] the arguments for giving priority to medical improvement in an overall colonial development policy were stepped up and buttressed with statistics aimed at alleviating the concerns of budget-minded critics. It appears that over a period of ten years the medical directors had not only perfected their arguments but had also convinced themselves that development must be pursued and that a new approach to preventive medicine must be worked out. The proposed training school could prevent the waste of infant and adult life. One-quarter to one-half of infants born died within one year. Comparable data for England at that time showed a remarkable decline of infant deaths from one-sixth in 1870 to one-twentieth in 1939. With an average population density of only 14 per one square mile, Tanganyika could not permit its population to be wasted before it reached the age of only one year.[13] Thus, as in early colonial days, the spending of money to save lives was justified as a potential asset in any development plan because it would save money in the long run, even if a precise value could not be placed on a single life.

At this time, sufficient information had been gathered over the years to present a solid and comprehensive health plan.[14] Why then was the system ineffective? The major reason was the medical department's inability to distribute its staff more evenly in order to implement the social goals of the general development plan. Since the expansion of the medical services depended on increased revenue, little could be done within the foreseeable future. In 1939, 11 percent of the recurrent expenditure was allotted for the medical department, a percentage which the medical director considered insufficient.[15] The choice was to leave things as they were or to change from a predominantly European staff to a predominantly African auxiliary staff, an unrealistic goal in 1939. It is doubtful whether contemporary opinion was ready to accept an interpretation of medical services as not necessarily revenue producing. It did not help to point out that a part of the money spent on medicine was retrieved through "invisible" returns by better labor productivity as the result of better health. It was also said that some of the "visible" returns of the medical services could not be measured in terms of immediate profit but only "in the shape of lives, especially infant lives, saved."[16]

In spite of ten years of delays, the medical administration submitted still another set of suggestions to the Development Committee of 1939. Among the more important proposals was a new request for a tuberculosis hospital, a central unit which would serve to isolate patients. But equally important as the isolation of infective patients would be a broad and rigid system of education for the sick and the healthy. Through education, through constant reminders of the dangers of the threat of infection to the lives of the sick as well as their families, the natives were to be weaned of customs which contributed to infection and disease. The "dangerous native customs," caused by fear of raids or theft, consisted in having the entire family with all their movable possessions under one roof. The situation was aggravated by fear of night and night air and "the complete ignorance of the method of transmission of infectious disease." The natives (the report said) "have a faculty for the appreciation of logic which is not greatly inferior to that of the white races, but as in those white races, for logic to be of value, it must be based on the conviction that the premises on which the logic depends are irrefutably true." For that purpose, the whole system of education must be directed toward securing benefit to the African. Similar statements had been made in England during the mid-nineteenth century. The Chadwickian health apostles, however, had used compulsion to lead the errant and ignorant Englishmen to the gospel of health and sanitation. In colonial Tanganyika, in the 1930s and 1940s, coercion in the interest of public health was not to be used. One hoped to combat tuberculosis by "explaining" to the Africans what the nature of infectious tuberculosis was and by convincing them of the rationality of the advocated measures. One had confidence in the ability of an untrained mind to learn by experience and by example.[17]

The medical department's philosophy and its reasoning on development were often ambiguous during this period of changing attitudes. The department favored the expansion of social services if they could be paid for, and occasionally made exceptions for vital projects even where local funds were scarce.[18] Since the Acts of 1940 and 1945 added the promotion of welfare to the theme of development, some of the ambiguities in development thinking had to yield to more precise definitions of the ultimate objectives. It is interesting to observe that the objectives of the early 1920s and 1930s are repeated, confirmed, and explained throughout the 1940s, but there is a greater sense of urgency. It is no longer necessary to explain why sixty doctors cannot cope with several millions of Africans and why 120 doctors are considered the minimum.

By 1942 medicine was described as a link in "the chain of social services" together with agriculture, husbandry, forestry, soil conservation, and better education which were equally vital in development-oriented programs.[19] The quality of medical services, it was said, must be freed from their dependence on economic fluctuations, expanding during periods of prosperity and retrenching during depressions, as had happened over the years between 1920 and 1940. When Dr. E. D. Pridie, Chief Medical Officer of the Colonial Office, visited Tanganyika in 1949, he was shocked by the shortage of doctors in the colony and attributed it to the absorption of British doctors in the British National Health Services after World War II.[20] He saw only one way out, and that was the immediate training of African staff to relieve the professional medical personnel–not a new idea. Would it remain an empty postulate or would the training of Africans finally be started in earnest?

The Medical Department's proposals for development in 1944 were not substantially different from those of 1930, except that the reduction of staff for the purpose of economizing was rejected. Dr. Scott called for "reinforcement [of the service] in the shape of finance, drive, energy," plus the raising of the standard of living of the African population, whose standard made it impossible as yet to contribute financially to the service.[21]

The entry of Dr. P. A. T. Sneath on the scene in 1945 injected new life into the discussion on general development and its application to medical matters. After two years as director of the Tanganyika medical services, he had very definite views on the future of medical policy in an impoverished country with a large population of which only a fraction could be reached by the medical personnel in 1947. He expressed his views in several memoranda to the Provincial Commissioner and to the Secretary of Government in Dar es Salaam. He evaluated native rural services, tribal dressers, and the dispensary system from the perspective of the concerned professional doctor dedicated to the principles and standards of western medicine.[22] He faced several major problems head on: he had to deal with the shortage of medical manpower, and he had to satisfy the Provincial Administration's desire to give immediate and tangible relief to rural communities. Finally, he had to dispel the suspicion that as a medical professional he was at odds with the ever-growing demand for local native dispensaries.

In his carefully prepared analysis of public health in Tanzania, submitted to the Provincial Commissioners' Conference in 1947, he outlined the history of tribal dispensaries since 1926.[23] Sneath was an important link between the slow-moving pace of medicine during the twenties and thirties, and the more adventurous approaches of the 1950s.

In 1947, when Sneath submitted new proposals for the future of medical policy in Tanzania, he described himself as handicapped by a misinterpretation of his views. He was not "politically and practically retrograde," as apparently his non-professional colleagues described him. There seemed to be an unavoidable conflict between the medical professional attempting not to sacrifice quality of medical service, and the provincial administrator who favored immediate action in curative and preventive medicine for the masses of the rural population.[24] The conflict between the guardian of medical quality and the provincial administrator concerned with the political and social impact of medical aid was not new, but the need for action was more acute after World War II.

Sneath saw two alternatives. Government could either alleviate individual cases of illness temporarily throughout the country with the aid of untrained personnel, or it would provide quality service stretching it to the utmost limits, fully aware that medical aid could only reach clusters of people who lived within reach of properly supervised health stations. The question, then, was whether the interests of thousands of sick people and others exposed to disease could be sacrificed, even if only temporarily, or whether the interests of large groups near population centers must come first. He dismissed as hypocritical the pretension that government could supply services for the entire population at a time when it did not have enough trained African assistants.[25]

In a lengthy memorandum on a history of the tribal dresser system in Tanzania, he gave full credit to the merit of the principle, but he objected to the shoddy quality that the service had reached so far because it had given priority to political considerations and had neglected to construct a firm basis for a system of African dispensers. Instead, it had started the program with youth whose educational level was unacceptable, with school leavers unable to absorb the essential elementary training in the sciences in order to become medical assistants. He also felt that the sudden change from their accustomed cultural environment to their new tasks as medical assistants left them unprepared to assume the discipline and responsibilities of their medical jobs. They became, he wrote, half-trained assistants, with a sham confidence in their abilities, and did more harm than good over the years. He cited the example of Lake Province, where, in 1943, 90 percent of the newly-trained assistants were "useless from the medical point of view, having quite naturally degenerated from the effect of their surroundings into dishonest and incapable practitioners."[26] Harsh words indeed, at a time when young Africans made education and participation in government one of their major goals. It must be remembered, however, that Sneath held the Administration–and not the young Africans–responsible for the shortcomings.

Did he have a remedy? Sneath favored a gradual expansion of an outreach medical service. He spoke of an intensive network from which auxiliary services should radiate as time went on. The time element was essential in 1950, however, and arguments for or against quality service first and extension services later could be continued endlessly depending upon one's point of view. Sneath persevered, saying, "this type of [slow] development might be thought hard upon the more remote sections of the population, but was considered to be the only sound means of developing the rural service as a whole. It would eventually, in fairness, have to be maintained at least in part from central funds."[27]

Sneath's report to Secretary of Government in Dar es Salaam came at a time when the overall achievements of the development plans in East Africa were critically evaluated. This was the time for Lord Hailey to have his original African Survey of 1938 reviewed and revised from a new perspective. Was Sneath just a stickler for standards which were not attainable in Tanzania in 1950, or did he represent the transition to a new approach in the 1950s? The latter seems to be true, as Dr. E. D. Pridie's "Review of the Medical Policy of Tanganyika" in November 1949 clearly indicates.[28]

Government contributions for medical development up to this point are not impressive.[29] Apart from statistics, however, the changing attitudes toward spending on social development reflect the new thinking in terms of African development. In the revised development plan for Tanganyika for the years 1950-1956, a "remarkably rapid general development since the end of World War II" is acknowledged. In fact, the development of natural resources, increased mining activities, and a considerable increase of commercial and industrial activities influenced the decision to review and revise the earlier ten-year development plan after only three years of its course. Priorities were to be reconsidered. The emphasis originally placed on communications, namely £13,785,000 out of a total budget of £36,411,000, reflected the conventional preference of material development; or, as stated in the report, the priority given to economic and productive development.[30] Social services were to be increased–though budgeted for only £3 million (almost £2 million less than in 1946)–because the Territorial contribution for the services had been increased. The medical development was to include as its biggest item a new African hospital in Dar es Salaam and minor medical buildings throughout the Territory, but no provisions for rural services were made, apparently because they were considered part of the general budget. It may also have been assumed that the expansion of rural medical services required too many basic changes in education and training to be included in a program of only five years.

In the light of these figures, can one still speak of a change of attitude? I believe that the 1945 ten-year Colonial Development Plan and its revision of 1949 point in a new direction by emphasizing the long-term commitment of funds and by expressly including social issues, even though they were not sufficiently funded. Planning for education and preventive medicine—previously forced to yield to goals set for communications, water supplies, and natural resources—was firmly put on record. With the extension of development planning from five-year periods to ten-year periods, the implementation of the needs of elementary education could be undertaken more realistically. Critics will point out that the beginning of social improvements, coming as late as 1956 (only five years before the independence of Tanzania), was not impressive because it was too little, too late. Seen historically, however, a great difference existed between the official view of the 1920s—when colonial development was described as a means to relieve unemployment in Britain[31]—and the official view in 1947, when "raising the standard of living [of the African] by industrial development" was given the close attention of colonial governments.[32]

3

RURAL MEDICAL SERVICES: THE COLONIAL PERIOD

In the preceding chapter, the rural medical services were described as playing a minor role in development planning before independence in Tanzania. Though the notion was accepted that rural dispensaries were the key to preventive medicine, social change, and economic growth, many of the schemes for the expansion of rural treatment centers were not implemented. The reasons for failing to do so are complex and shall be presented in the present chapter.

In 1926, yielding to popular demand and political pressure, the colonial administration agreed to establish rural dispensaries.[1] This decision was in line with the philosophy of indirect rule adopted in Tanganyika after the British had become the Mandatory Power of the Territory under the League of Nations. A dispensary system staffed by Africans seemed to be the answer to the problem of insufficient manpower, the shortage of funds for administrative purposes, and the general trend toward liberalizing colonial services.[2] Provincial officials considered the desire by Native Authorities to introduce their own tribal dressing stations as proof of the success of western medicine. Whereas before World War I the problem of how to "sell" the blessings of western medicine to Africans had been a major concern to many medical administrators, the opposite seemed to be true after 1918. In the 1920s, colonial officials asked themselves how to slow down the erratic growth of native tribal dispensaries.[3]

How can one explain this change? Until World War I, the original reason for the establishment of colonial medical services was adhered to rather rigidly. As late as 1922, Dr. John Gilks, new Principal Medical Officer (PMO) in Kenya, described preventive medical work in the early days as maintenance in a sanitary condition of small administrative stations serving a population of half a dozen Europeans and perhaps fifty or a hundred native troops or police. With the opening of the Uganda railway and greater mobility of medical officers, the 1913-14 estimates made provision for one PMO, one Deputy PMO, and one Sanitary Officer. In 1918, the Medical Department was permitted to add ten medical officers of health. By 1922, Gilks wrote:

> The Medical Department as a whole was no longer considered merely as an organization maintained by Government to facilitate administration by maintaining the personnel of the executive in health, but as a Department of Government responsible for the carrying out of the most important function for which Government itself is established, namely the maintenance in health of the general population of the country and the improvement of the conditions under which that population lives.[4]

From this forceful 1922 recognition of the needs and rights of the masses of peasants in East Africa to the first piece of legislation setting up rural dispensaries in 1926, the change in the concept of what medicine should do in Africa might almost be called radical; while the long time that elapsed between 1926 and the realization of a functional system of rural medicine in 1946 (however inadequate as yet) appears unconscionable and invites criticism.

Recent writers on the subject have, indeed, been critical of a colonial administration that did not act more expeditiously on the establishment of rural medical services. If one bases the analysis of medical improvements primarily on economic data, that is, the funds spent on European hospitals and the money allotted to Native Treasuries from central funds, the criticism is justified. Other factors must be considered, however. There were the on-going debates within the medical department, the provincial administration, and the advisory boards in London, which had to be considered. There was also the actual status of Native Authority government, not its ideal model that existed only in the minds of planners. There were the cultural disparities between African traditions and European concepts which any evaluation of rural medicine must include to comprehend the complex nature of that part of medical history and African development.[5]

It is worth noting that in 1922, when the general debate on colonial development barely began to take shape in Britain, Dr. Gilks, the medical administrator in Kenya, had come independently to the conclusion that the promotion of better living conditions for the entire population in his realm of Kenya was essential. From his point of view, therefore, it was not an about-face move at all to accept dispensaries as an arm of the central health authority in 1926. That was not enough, however. With hardly a medical staff in its central administration, Native Authorities could not instantly recruit the trained young Africans they needed. This was known to Government. That it accepted the expansion of medicine through rural dispensaries—though they were not yet operable at the time when they were established—seems to indicate that Government considered this development as inevitable in the future. There were from the outset three different segments of government that dealt with the same problem from a different perspective and with different degrees of determination. There was the Medical Department, changing its views on professionalism and social philosophy over the years. There was the Provincial Administration, especially in Tanzania, influenced by political and social considerations in its relations with the African population. Finally, there were the authorities in England, who were susceptible to shifting views on general colonial administration. This is one of the causes for the many setbacks of the developments of rural dispensaries between 1926 and 1956.

The bare outline of the history of rural dispensaries since 1926 shows these and other conflicting trends. Until 1930, the dispensaries seemed to thrive without much effort. Simple wattle and daub huts with one, two, or three rooms were set up and maintained by Native Authorities. The medical department's role was purely advisory. Selected youths were trained for three months and the territorial administration was responsible for matters of discipline and administration. Depending on whether one judges the performance of Native Authority (NA) rural dispensaries from Provincial Officers' reports or from those of the medical administration in Kenya and Tanzania, a different picture will emerge. From 1926, when the dispensaries started, to 1933 when the Depression limited funds for East African budgets, provincial reports exude optimism. In Tanganyika, from Central Province, and from Iringa as well as Mwanza, for instance, attendance at dispensaries during the first four years since 1926 was described as good. NA's were quoted as constantly opening new ones. Dispensaries were popular and given "good marks," as in Central Province, for example, where they were rated as doing valuable and efficient work, capable of dealing with ulcers, jiggers, and local maladies. Africans expressed confidence in their dressers and chiefs, and even praised the European doctors who had the overall responsibility. The Provincial Commissioner of Central Province quoted chiefs in the area as full of pride in their "great native hospital in Dodoma" and reported their remark that "truly a sick man is a sick man, whether he is black or white."[6] It seems that there was sufficient supervision by medical officers in this district. Apparently anticipating criticism by the Medical Department, the Commissioner of Central Province added in his 1933 report the following statement, which is quite typical of the Provincial Administration's attitude toward dispensaries:

> In moving the Native Authorities to set up these dispensaries the layman has had to rely on his personal observation as to apparent results in the general health and to fortify himself with the reflection that, if dispensaries simply supply clean bandages and a safety pin to take the place of filthy rags, their establishment is well worth while.[7]

The varying and incomplete statistics in the official reports do not give an accurate account of dispensaries in operation during the first decade. Starting with zero tribal dressers in 1926, their number reached 90 in 1927, climbed to 147 in 1928, and peaked at 288 in 1930, with a total attendance of new cases in the same year of 352,423 Africans.[8] For a total population estimated for Tanganyika Territory at 7.5 million at the time, the number is not impressive; as an indication of the acceptance of the rural services by Africans and their leaders, however, it confirms the views of those administrators who supported dispensaries as a political weapon.

If one listens to a story told by the central medical department in Tanzania, the response is less promising. By 1933, with 303 tribal dressers actually working as rural medical assistants and taking care of peasant families not otherwise reached by doctors or their African trained assistants, it was discovered that the euphoria about the progress toward an all-encompassing spread of western medical aid was unfounded. The much-hoped-for "native public health service" was not yet on the horizon. According to the "History of the Tribal Dresser System" compiled in 1947, the system

> was in practice failing to fulfill even the elementary purpose for which it had first been intended. A few dressers were doing useful work, but the majority were overreaching themselves. Misdiagnosis was leading to wastage and sometimes even to positive harm, and figures returned did not give a true estimate of the work done owing to faking, frequent sampling of medicines, and general inaccuracy.[9]

In Lake Province, where dispensaries were better organized, nothing had been done to improve the skill and knowledge of the personnel. Therefore, endemic disease was not touched. It was not a lack of good intentions or the insufficiency of funds which was responsible for the shortcomings, according to the medical department's analysis, but the lack of supervision, the bad roads, and the remoteness of so many of the stations from the center in Dar es Salaam.

At the native hospital in Mwanza, a training station for dressers was set up to train and retrain dressers already working in the area. This, too, proved a failure because School Standard VIII as a prerequisite for training could not be secured.[10] The eighteen months' course of training at Mwanza was quite sophisticated: it included physics, anatomy, physiology, microscopic techniques, and diagnosis of some more frequent diseases such as ulcers, burns, eye infections, and contagious diseases. The course aimed in the right direction of basic technical training, but it ignored the prevalent absence of educational standards. The development funds between 1930 and 1940 had not been spent on education.

A reorganization of the rural services in Tanganyika began in 1935, but it was not completed by the outbreak of World War II, although the several training centers in Lake Province (as well as Western, Eastern, and Northern Provinces) operated with varying degrees of success. By 1941, the number of cases treated in NA stations had risen to "well over a million" annually.[11] As was seen before,[12] the medical administration blamed political motives of colonial government for the qualitatively poor services because it permitted NA's to expand too quickly. The transfer, however, of NA dispensaries to the medical department for guidance and supervision was rejected by the Territory's administration for the same reasons. It was considered important "to further the political education of the Native Authorities by allowing them control of their own social services."[13] In any case, it was a futile consideration because the Department of Medical and Sanitary Services did not have the money to pay for rural dispensaries. Mwanza remained the best training center in the interior and was even in a position to raise its entrance requirements to the as-yet highest educational level of Standard X. It also paid accordingly a high salary of 60 shillings per month to its assistants, and produced a superior group of trainees. On the whole, however, the educational and financial inequality among training schools and recruits continued. After World War II, one returned to the practice of a centrally directed rural service effectively supervised by a few developed medical centers. The remote rural areas continued with limited first-aid-type service. This, according to the judgment of the Territorial Administration, was the only way of developing a rural service (which was, of course, a contradiction in itself, because it included only areas where population density, tax structures, and existing hospital facilities served a limited number of satellite rural facilities).[14]

By 1949, the see-saw battle for or against a system of rural medical services appeared to approach a compromise. A subcommittee deliberating on the future of rural medical services expressed its views this way: "In the past their [medical men] bias has been very largely toward curative work as was inevitable considering their development from a service to maintain immigrant Government Officers in Health." There was, the sub-committee wrote, a difference between western Europe and the colonies, and to apply European methods was responsible for the failure to eradicate community-wide diseases. Not enough was done, they concluded, "on account of the historical beginnings of the service and on account of the desire of the indigenous population to participate in a similar service."[15] They recommended that a health service along new lines be established.

The final recommendations submitted to the full committee on the future of rural medical services in 1948 set up two categories of rural medical aid stations, Grades A and B. Grade A was to include and upgrade all stations within a thirty-mile range of either government or mission medical officers. Grade B was to be reduced to first-aid functions for which the Medical Department did not assume responsibility. This recommendation bears the imprint of P. E. T. Sneath's opposition to substandard medical practices. After Dr. Pridie, Chief Medical Officer of the Colonial Office, visited Tanganyika Territory in 1949, the report was set aside and replaced by a new set of guidelines issued as *Sessional Paper* by the Colonial Office. Though committed to the expansion of rural medicine, the new outline made government even more responsible for "constant" supervision of all rural medical stations. Central government and its representatives were to be obligated to their control. New rural dispensaries were, therefore, not to be opened until after personnel was available for their staffing and supervision. With a staff of only seventy-four registered doctors and fifty licensed practitioners in 1948, it was unlikely that rural dispensaries would be expanded during the life of the new economic development plan of 1950.[16]

Was the new plan a victory for the medical conservatives, or for the progressives in the provincial administration who placed political and social improvement on a par with medical-professional objectives? The Pridie-inspired Sessional Paper on rural dispensaries stressed the departure from past practices (i.e., before 1948) and pledged itself to new ideas in the 1950s. Abandoning the previously prevailing focus on curative medicine, it proposed a wider conception of environmental sanitation, hygiene, and prevention. It promised continued cooperation with Native Authorities, including their moral and financial encouragement, but within the framework of a definite policy for the integration of rural health stations within the Territorial Health Service.[17]

The immediate future for the expansion of rural dispensaries was not promising. It depended on too many steps which had to be taken before results could be achieved. The salaries of medical rural helpers needed upgrading to attract better applicants. The Provincial Commissioners recommended at their annual conference in 1951 to have Grade A and B dispensaries taken over by the Medical Department in order to facilitate better financing and more direct control. At the same time they envisaged a miniature rural health center headed by an African doctor which would serve a variety of purposes, including preventive care, the promotion of environmental sanitation, the nutritional side of medicine, and education and community-oriented social policies. The list of suggestions for this utopian ideal of a future rural health center sounds more like a blueprint for the rehabilitation of a modern western urban decaying neighborhood.[18]

The last ten years before independence saw only piecemeal changes and frequent reevaluations of plans for future policy. It was evident that medical and social improvements could not be carried out in isolation. They depended on comprehensive and integrated economic development planning. In this respect Tanganyika's Development and Welfare Plan for 1950-1956 yields interesting insights. It shows a great disparity in priorities. The budgets for education and medicine were smaller than during the preceding two years. While the social services had been given 16 percent of the total budget during 1947-1949, they were now reduced to 12 percent of the total for 1950-1956. The reduction was justified on the ground that the Territorial Government had assumed responsibility for recurrent expenditure. This meant an automatic stalling of rural expansion which depended on non-routine budget items for auxiliary training, for materials, and for the construction of buildings and roads in order to expand the network of dispensaries. Hospitals in or near urban centers in the more densely populated areas would be favored by the new system against the remote countryside, which had no professional staff nearby. Unfortunately, the countryside needed medical aid more than anywhere else. The countryside was where expansion ought to have been planned and provided for. The medical reports of Sneath, Pridie, and other medical officers in the field had frequently complained about the inability of the Native Authorities to pay for improvements out of their own tax income. They considered the weakness of NA budgets as one of the major obstacles to the construction of a network of rural medical stations. The new Five Year Plan, however, allotted the major share of the social services budget to capital expenditure, including one group hospital in Dar es Salaam and one in Mwanza, with minor amounts going to such miscellany as a mental hospital, a leprosy center, and a few smaller stations. Education funds were also restricted to capital projects for construction of school buildings; funds were not allocated for instruction, which was the most urgently needed factor in the training of medical rural assistants. The third item of the Social Services budget, called social development, included rural social development. It received only £169,000 for five years. This should not come as a surprise, since the 1950 Plan, like those that had preceded it, stated clearly that "economic and productive development should take prior place."

Native Councils and native local governments were praised for their contribution and their active participation in territorial development, which was interpreted as an act of emancipation from the tutelage of colonial government. The African, it was said, had recognized the value of self-help and did not "merely regard the provision of water as a gift from a benevolent Government."[19] But the selection of priorities in the Plan shows that rural areas would not be the major beneficiaries of the social services. Urban improvement had priority. To guarantee urban development in major towns, an organization for African housing under the Commissioner for Development was proposed. Urban slums must be cared for first, rural areas might come later.

In the 1950s, a major change in the socio-medical programs in Tanganyika was not anticipated. It was assumed that with "the marked increase of commercial and industrial activities in the Territory" since World War II, development was inevitable and that it was the obligation of government to keep its policy in harmony with the general trend of progress. With emphasis placed on the economic rather than the non-productive sphere of development, the social services in the Revised Plan of 1950 were reduced from 29.4 percent of the original Ten-Year Plan to 12.0 percent. Medical funds were to be used for hospital construction, maternity wings, leprosariums, a tuberculosis hospital and minor structures. The Plan's impact on preventive medicine was bound to be of minor importance. The attitude toward development spending was clearly expressed in the statement that

> the most careful consideration has been given to the totals made available for Medical and Education buildings, and the sums . . . to be spent in the period 1950-56 are considered to be as large as can reasonably be set aside in view of their non-productive nature, except in the very widest sense of the term.[20]

Medical progress during the development phase of the 1950s was measured in terms of improvements for medical buildings and in a more economic use of manpower. But the prevention of the wastage of lives was not an issue for immediate remedial action at that particular time.

Development strategy and medical progress in Kenya during the 1940s and 1950s showed a different pattern. Although the promotion of rural medicine was advocated, the course of action showed many variations. The medical administrators appealed repeatedly to the Colonial Office stressing the plight of the African peasant who was unable to use his land to his best advantage although he lived on relatively fertile soil. They also pointed at the insanitary conditions and the lack of education, responsible for the low level of civilization that the rural population endured. They saw evidence that the young people of Kenya did not lag in a desire for material prosperity or for better living conditions.[21] Dr. John L. Gilks, PMO in Nairobi between 1920 and 1931, and his successor Dr. A. R. Paterson, PMO between 1931 and 1941, represented these views.

Dr. Gilks recognized the necessity to reach the population outside of Nairobi. Local government in Kenya was different from that of Tanganyika. Local Native Councils, established in 1924, were directed by a District Commissioner. Headmen and other native officials were appointed as the governor saw fit. Local councils could recommend matters affecting local administration, if approved by the governor. The councils could pass resolutions on public health but this did not mean that the resolutions must be adopted by the headmen who were regarded as government employees and whose salary came from central revenues.[22] Nevertheless, Gilks was pleased with the interest that local councils showed in public health by voting for dispensaries. He found out, however, that this was not enough and complained in 1926 that "little impression had been made on native reserves by sanitary measures," and that sanitary precaution was not practiced.[23]

It was largely, however, the depression and the decline of medical estimates from £250,000 in 1931 to £200,000 in 1934 which prevented the expansion of

African dispensaries and caused concern to Gilks' successor, Dr. Paterson, in 1934. He continued the advocacy of European-staffed primary medical centers in the Reserves, and he favored secondary medical centers manned by only one or two "trained medical officers."[24] In spite of an imaginative conception of what ought to be done for the African population, however, his grasp of rural dispensaries was limited. He saw them as a vehicle for preventive sanitation and hence was resigned to their failure. How could a peasant with an annual family income of only £13 buy soap, install windows in his hut and have proper lighting and sufficient education to understand sanitary needs, when he would have needed a minimum of at least £18 to do so?

After World War II, a new policy of developing health centers in "native land units" was introduced. The centers were to serve several objectives. They should provide treatment in the homes of patients for "short-term fevers" and for illnesses that did not require hospitalization. More important, however, they should be instrumental in integrating preventive and promotional services with the help of an African team of a health assistant, a health visitor and a midwife. Their task would be to help educate the rural people in public health matters and sanitation. Always, however, it was stressed that such services were purely ancillary which presumably meant that the weight of medical services rested with the established medical institutions.[25] The rural health services continued to be run by local health authorities. The number of centers had risen to 19 in 1955, five years after their start in 1950.

Until Kenya's independence in 1963, the rural health centers suffered from a serious lack of financing and the administration's inability to train a sufficient number of medical aids for every center.[26] Local District Councils remained in charge of the centers although their weakness had been deplored over the years. Nevertheless, the much criticized centers held their own and even increased in numbers quite rapidly. There were 25 in 1957 and 140 in 1962, just before independence. Their growth was attributed to their popularity with the African population but the Ministry of Health also took credit for their growth from nil in 1946 to 140 in 1962.[27]

Geography, demography and the politics of settlement in Kenya gave the promotion of rural health a different character from that of Tanganyika whose population was thinly spread over a far larger land area. The fact that Britain began to rule Tanganyika in 1919, at a time when Kenya had been a colony for 34 years, influenced its colonial policy. Kenya was a colony with an influential element of white settlers whose views on rural development were clearly heard. Humanitarian and progressive ideas, even if not adopted, had an influence on the reports by Drs. Sneath and Pridie in Dar es Salaam between 1948 and 1951.[28] The issue of rural development in Kenya was seen primarily as a mandate for the medical service, charged with the responsibility of fulfilling a task delegated to it by the home government. Individual medical directors understood the urgency to give medical aid to the rural population, but the debates on the subject were carried on in a less emotional way and with much less moralizing. Another factor, not present in Tanganyika, was introduced in Kenya in the early 1950s when the Mau Mau unrest required protection in the rural areas near Nairobi. It coincided with the beginning of the expansion of rural medicine in Kenya. The colonial administration established concentrated settlements in Kikuyu Province near Nairobi in order to protect Kenyan peasants from Mau Mau attacks. Peasants gathered in these regrouped villages required different treatment from those in outlying areas.

In spite of these and other internal troubles in the 1950s, rural medicine in Kenya was affected by the Colonial Development and Welfare Plans after 1945. Spending on medical services increased steadily and with it came new commitments, such as the demand for social services and the improvement of the quality of medical services. Spending on medical services was increased. It rose from £360,000 in 1945 to £2,602,832 in 1962. The indivisibility of the health services was accepted in principle which meant that a large share of funds must be allocated to preventive measures while the curative services must progress simultaneously. How these objectives could be maintained will be discussed in another chapter.

4

RESEARCH AND DEVELOPMENT: THE COLONIAL PERIOD

Medicine was one of several factors which played a vital role in the development of colonial East Africa. Increasingly, its direct impact on economics, politics, society and internal administration was felt more keenly and the need for scientific research in medicine and related areas was recognized. One is tempted to compare the difference of pace in the development of research in science, agriculture, anthropology and demography in nineteenth and early twentieth century Europe with the relative suddenness with which problems requiring research erupted in tropical eastern Africa. The problems of preventive and curative medicine and their dependence on environmental factors demanded objective analyses and scientific investigations from the beginning of colonial penetration in Africa, even though they occurred in a historical situation very different from the western world. In spite of the universality of the scientific method, the role it played in colonial East Africa, however, shows great differences. The presentation of a few landmarks in the emergence of scientific research in colonial East Africa will serve as an illustration of its unique impact on man and society in Kenya and Tanzania.[1]

Colonial administrators were aware from the outset of the dangers which climate, disease and geography posed to their own lives and to the lives of Africans. They admitted their fears in this respect and expressed their concern about the seemingly insurmountable problems which they faced in trying to transplant elements of western agriculture and industry to tropical Africa. At first they identified their doubts as merely the problem of the "unknown." They were concerned about the hazardous nature of their venture to plan even a simple system of control over "the dark forces of nature" and the containment of disease in man, cattle and crops. The need for research to advance their knowledge was stressed as early as 1900, but the East African Bureau of Research in Medicine and Hygiene, established to finance and coordinate research, was not set up in Nairobi until 1949. Why did it take so long?

Early in the century, the Royal Society in London, the originator of research programs, became alarmed when malaria and other tropical diseases spread in the colonies. In 1903, Sir Michael Foster, the Secretary of the Society, urged that in order to safeguard the prosperity of the empire in tropical countries, a permanent organization for the study of the nature of prevention "might fairly be expected to furnish an adequate return for money spent on it." Joseph Chamberlain supported the allocation of funds from the Tropical Diseases Research Fund in London and expected modest contributions from the colonies themselves. The success of the scheme depended on the maintenance of a link between England and the colonial practioners. And that link was tenuous for a long time.

While England itself was becoming statistically-minded during the first decade of the twentieth century, reliable statistics for the colonies were either not collected, or if they were, they were not available for interpretation. Comparative data on tropical disease, population fluctuations and infant mortality, though reported by medical departments, went to waste as far as research was concerned. Equally important was the basic attitude which related investment in science in the colonies to the retrieval of money not spent for productive purposes. Alfred Milner, Colonial Secretary in 1919, regretted that opportunities in the colonies were lost in spite of the great opportunities they offered. "There is no better investment for the money of any Colony than scientific research, both medical and economic," Milner said to the Special Committee of Inquiry on the Colonial Medical Services.[2]

In 1928, Dr. John L. Gilks extended the interpretation of the value of organized and subsidized research beyond the economic perspective. As director of medical services in Kenya, he described malaria as a social disease which was aggravated by a low standard of living among the bulk of the population. This opened up a new approach to disease. If the general standard of living was to be improved, research into medical as well as social factors must be conducted and coordinated. Scientific research extended its focus to the related factors of living conditions of Africans, to the treatment of labor and the role of native custom in public health policy. In the future, scientific research into health problems would have to include a vastly expanded range of factors which would later directly influence programs of development in the 1950s.[3]

In 1934, Dr. A. R. Paterson, medical director in Kenya after Dr. Gilk's retirement, extended the range of objectives that might be served by research. He spoke of research to serve the development of the peoples in the colony through a better knowledge of social, environmental and biological factors. He proposed research into the psychological and psychiatric conditions of prisoners. He also suggested research into the special conditions that triggered malignant diseases in East Africa. The suggestions were broad and general, but they indicate a new approach to the concept of development in Africa.

During the next twenty years, progress was limited to the level of organization. In the minds of professional men, administrators and political leaders, medicine, research and development were interdependent. A research organization in the East African colonies began to evolve very slowly, after having rested on the drawing boards in the 1940s and early 1950s.[4] A Conference on Research agreed in 1936 to set up a standing medical research committee but it was kept in limbo during the Second World War. After an exhaustive investigation of research conditions in East Africa by Professor E. A. McSwinney of St. Thomas Hospital in London, the establishment of a Bureau of Health was recommended in 1947 with funds of £5,000 annually from the Colonial Development and Welfare Fund. It finally led to the foundation of an East African Bureau of Research in Medicine and Hygiene in 1949 and the creation of an interterritorial Advisory Committee on Medical Research in East Africa in 1952. The Bureau operated under the East African High Commission which had just been established in 1948, formalizing the de facto integration of the East African administrative services under one central authority. From here on, the Bureau gradually established its priorities, only to be placed under the East African Community in 1961.[5]

Dr. E. B. Worthington, first Scientific Secretary of the East Africa High Commission, was an influential booster of research and scientific services in East Africa. Contrary to the cautious recommendations of his predecessors, he demanded the paramountcy of science and scientific research in tropical East Africa. He found that a great deal of development in East Africa had taken place in the wrong way, unduly expensive because there was insufficient knowledge to go on, or because it was not available at all. He demanded that research be given a central role. That was in 1956.[6] During the last years of the colonial administration in Kenya and Tanzania, with an eye on the impending political changes, the basis of a central research structure had finally been completed. Under the East African Community and its Research Council after 1961, economic and social development was emphasized and its dependence on scientific research was stressed by the new governments. It is paradoxical that this was done at a time when the new national governments were hardly in a position to invest time, energy and their sparse funds in research. But the incorporation of research in science and medicine in the basic economy of tropical Africa was a valuable legacy bequeathed by the colonial powers to their "wards."

It would be historically incorrect not to give credit to the specific achievements of disease control in the area of epidemiology and disease in general. Campaigns against trypanosomiasis were done under the direction of researchers and with the aid of teams of doctors. Research in chemistry, zoology, biology and infectious disease, performed outside Africa, contributed to the record of prevention in Africa. What Worthington and other critics stressed is the fact that action was taken after an emergency instead of five years in advance of an outbreak.

This is not the place to evaluate the medical record of colonial medicine.[7] It is the continuity of the history of research in relation to development that has been examined in this chapter. The need for a research organization which would secure sufficient funds for research was fully appreciated between 1930 and 1960 but it was not implemented in the system as a whole until 1949, and it did not become effective until close to the end of the colonial period.[8]

Furthermore, the efforts of men like Robert Koch and Ronald Ross (1898 and 1903), Sir David Bruce and others in trypanosomiasis research (1903), the treatment of tuberculosis among Africans during the colonial period, to cite just a few examples here, are proof that individuals or departments of government reacted immediately in medical and epidemiological emergencies by researching the cause of the outbreak and by taking preventive and remedial action if possible as circumstances allowed. But in isolation and cut off from resources even when given emergency funds from the London government, they could not chart a course for future development. The resettlement policy in the struggle against trypanosomiasis began in 1903 and continued into the interwar period. It is a good example of the interdepartmental approach necessitated by the struggle against tsetse. From the treatment of patients in large camps, it expanded to large-scale tree cutting operations in the bush, the relocation in "clean" settlements, special efforts to reduce tribal resistance to resettlement in unfamiliar locations considered to be safe by government but not always liked by the peasants, and demonstration programs of new agricultural methods. In fact, the control of trypanosomiasis was the most striking example of the use of government-subsidized scientific research in eastern Africa.

Closely related to research in medicine was research in agriculture which culminated in R. J. M. Swynnerton's project presented in 1953 as "A Plan to Intensify the Development of African Agriculture in Kenya."[9] Written at a time of Mau Mau unrest among the Kikuyu, it was an investigation into the causes of Kikuyu dissatisfaction over land alienation in the Kenya Highlands. It took a bold step ahead in rethinking the existing pattern of land use by African peasants and suggesting a more profitable method of more intensive agricultural production and reorganization of landownership. The intensive plan, as proposed in 1953, was to extend over a five-year period from 1955 to 1960. It investigated the Kikuyu traditional pattern of landownership, it examined the reasons for the low output of agricultural production, it stressed the fatal consequences of overgrazing and it proposed the training of Africans in the use of more rational methods of potentially profitable crops without necessarily having to depend on imported modern technology. In this respect, it was radically innovative, anticipating similar ideas in today's rural program of agriculture in Tanzania.

Swynnerton was not a romantic dreamer. He knew that mere suggestions to Africans to use better methods of cultivation were not enough. He proposed demonstration programs, constant supervision, training to reach the goal of producing cash crops for the small African peasant in the interest of improving his health. A particular delicate problem was the issue of land tenure and inheritance of land, because the best land was in the hands of the settlers and because land inheritance practices led to fragmentation of small parcels and could not be intensively and economically used. Such changes required cooperation by the owners and the subsequent changes in titles had to go through the courts. Although Swynnerton was aware of the preliminary problems which had to be overcome, he saw the proposed five-year agricultural development plan as the essential prerequisite in the interest of the nonwestern sector of the economy of Kenya and in the interest of the general health of the population.

The proposal incorporated scientific research into crop production, nutrition, social custom, and political custom. Swynnerton's proposals revealed a missionary zeal similar to that of the medical personnel in the 1930s. In recommending agricultural education as one of the tools to effect change, he proposed to include African farmers, their children at school, and their teachers. He recommended the use of African administrators and African cooperative societies as opinion-makers. He proposed intensified investigations into soils, fertilizers and crop pests. He reminded the government that the success of the plan depended as much on people in high positions as on the energy of officers who had to implement it.

As was noticed in the history of the East African Medical Research Council introduced in the 1950s, the plan for intensive agricultural development came toward the end of the colonial period. We shall see later how it was implemented after the end of colonial government.

Nutrition was another issue that required scientific investigation if it was to influence development in eastern Africa. Discussed by colonial medical administrators, it could not really become an effective program without access to African families and their way of life.

In his statement on the state of health of the native population in 1926, Dr. Gilks described the native as "still living and dying under age-long conditions of insanitation." How could nutrition become an issue under these circumstances? Gilks knew that his department with a handful of medical officers could not have an impact on their lives. "Sickness and death, the result of poor nutrition, poor housing, harmful habits and customs, and complete lack of sanitary precaution, remain uncontrolled."[10] At this early stage, food habits and better nutrition were described as entirely dependent on the African's will to change his customary way of life. Such a change could not occur without education and training.

In 1936, Dr. A. R. Paterson, like Gilks a medical director in Kenya, came to almost the same conclusion. He thought progress depended on the people themselves since a small sanitary staff could not influence their lives. To improve the quality of their lives, they themselves must determine to do so.[11] It appears that neither changes in nutrition nor research in nutrition did have a place in African affairs before World War II.

A slow change came with the foundation of the East African Medical Survey and Research Institute in 1954. Instead of giving up hope of penetrating to the root of African habits under the prevailing conditions, the Institute commissioned a survey to collect data on the African school child and the family in which it lived. The survey presented at least a basis for further statistical analysis. The work did not always progress smoothly because of " ignorance and superstition" in a number of households. But a volume of information was collected on the day-to-day conditions of life among six widely-differing peoples in Tanzania. The surveyors succeeded in presenting for the first time a dietary survey and a report on infant malnutrition.[12]

The relationship between nutrition and development, however, would have to be defined on a broader basis. As long as development analysts assessed development primarily in terms of economic goals, nutrition would not be given priority as an important factor in the improvement of the quality of life of the population, except in its impact on greater labor productivity. Michael Latham pointed out in a paper "Priorities for Nutrition and Health Programs in Africa" that

> a lowered disease incidence, a better nourished population, an improved infant and toddler mortality rate are perhaps better indicators of development than national averages of telephones or automobiles per 1000 families, or even than dollars or shillings per capita.[13]

The dependence of labor productivity on nutrition was recognized early in the 19th century without connecting it in any way with development. Sorokin referred to the 19th century slave-owners in Brazil to whom malnutrition meant reduced economic returns. They therefore saw to it that their black slaves were the best-nourished group.[14]

We have seen that research in pure science and its application to the medical, social, economic and political condition in eastern Africa between 1946 and 1963 added a new factor in planning under the colonial administration. But it was only a beginning. New priorities after independence set different goals which gave research a different direction. It was important, however, that the basis for scientific research had been established, that its dependence on financial support had been demonsatrated and that its existence had been justified regardless of whether tangible results could be achieved in the immediate future.

5

TRANSITION TO INDEPENDENCE AND THE CONTINUITY OF MEDICAL GOALS

The planning for development in eastern Africa in the 1950s was influenced by subtle and conflicting policy considerations in London and in Africa which were further complicated by economic and administrative needs of the territories. Colonial budgets reflected goals of economic growth but the juggling for priorities by those concerned with education, public health and agriculture showed the presence of political motives as well. "Priorities had to be altered," said the introduction to the revised development and welfare plan for 1950-1956, "in order to conform with the general trend of economic and social development of natural resources."[1] It listed African housing in addition to township development and social services among other more conventional items. Larger appropriations were needed because of commercial and industrial expansion. Other items, however, represented a greater concern with the living conditions of the African population. Ultimately, the choice of objectives for the 1950-1956 Plan represented a compromise of different schools of thought.[2]

Lord Hailey, for instance, had advocated long-range planning for development after World War II as a necessary step forward in colonial affairs. He had placed emphasis on schemes to promote the welfare of the colonial peoples which he considered as a necessary investment in terms of social, rather than economic, advance.[3] Sir Eric Pridie, the innovative planner for the improvement of medical services in the early 1950s, thought along similar lines when he advocated narrowing the gap between medical care in hospitals and the inadequate medical facilities for the vast majority of the peasants in rural areas.[4] More liberal thinkers in the Colonial Office in London, such as Sir Andrew Cohen and Creech Jones, defended their policy of preparing the colonies for a more immediate transition to independence, regardless of whether a substantial segment of the population had reached a certain level of education which was judged an essential prerequisite for independence. Such views, however, were not shared by some of the governors in Kenya and Tanganyika during the critical period between 1955 and 1960. Governors Mitchell and Twining stuck to the old principle of paternalism according to which it was the duty of the protecting power to civilize those who had not yet reached the enlightened stage in which self-government could be applied.[5]

Differences of views in London and in the administrative centers in East Africa slowed down the formulation of a program of transition acceptable to all sides. Sir Andrew Cohen was not perturbed by these differences. He even welcomed the frequent exchange of views between London and the colonial capitals. He found that direct contact between officials in different parts of the empire helped to maintain a balance between local initiative by governors and central direction from London.[6]

At the same time, important developments were taking place on another level. The Tanganyika African National Union (TANU) fought successfully for recognition as the major representative of Africans in local and district government. By 1958, TANU had won the right to present candidates for district councils and ultimately also for the Legislative Council. Their success influenced the Colonial Office in advancing the timetable for independence, and this again led to changes of strategy in the governor's office. In his analysis of political stratgies in Tanzania in the 1950s, Cranford Pratt has shown how TANU tipped the balance in favor of a speedier transfer of power from colonial dependence to national independence. The elections of 1958 which gave TANU a majority over other African parties and insured its members seats on the ministerial council did not present a problem to middle-level British provincial and district officials. They were interested in the continuation of their agricultural development programs during the transition and needed the willing cooperation by African peasants. This was especially important in schemes for stepped-up education which again was essential for success in the training of African health assistants in rural districts. Like Nyerere, TANU's leader, they favored the transfer of power without violence, which would allow the development plans to continue after 1961.[7]

Throughout these years of delicate maneuvering, the medical department seemed to continue its regular work without paying too much attention to the general political atmosphere. In 1956, it drafted its five-year plan without reference to potential political changes. It assumed that medical policy must continue without interruption. In its draft outline for 1956-1961, it listed the steady flux of territorial revenue as one uncertain factor which might affect its performance. But from the medical point of view, it stressed continuity. It used Pridie's report as a base line and pointed to 1961 as a target. It interpreted its role as the bearer of a tradition which, with proper funds, effort and good will, was bound to lead to a better future.

Let us briefly analyze its assumptions. It found Pridie's recommendations implemented in 1956 but admitted that much was still to be done. When the planners spoke of the implementation of Pridie's objectives in 1956, one can only interpret their statement as meaning that they were in agreement with the principle of a balanced development of preventive and curative services, but beyond that, the actual apportionment of funds to the two services precluded their own assumptions. There was more to it, however, than economic arguments. The writers of the report were not convinced that the country was ready to accept prevention. In spite of all the assertions that the medical department was ready and willing to take concrete steps to develop preventive and rural medical services, they believed that such a step was premature. Curative services, they said, was what the people understand and what they want—and, they continued, as in African conditions at present, preventive medicine can only hope to be accepted by the people through curative services, it is proposed to devote by far the greater part of the capital sum available from development sources to expansion of the hospital services.[8] This kind of argument was decisive in handing over to the new government in 1961 a hospital-centered medical system. But it should not be characterized as proof of rejection of the new trend toward prevention as stated by Pridie. The 1956 report is an example of the long historical process in colonial medical development, in the course of which better and more encompassing medical services were often proposed without being matched to the prevailing economic, political and social reality of the day.[9] The gospel of social medicine was proposed as early as 1920 and picked up periodically between 1920 and 1950, only to be stalemated again by external conditions, conflicting medical philosophies and colonial fiscal policies. As recent writers like to point out, it lacked a coherent ideological base. The historian, however, will not be satisfied with this interpretation which takes the events out of their historical context.

The 1956 Plan assigned the largest capital outlay to the new general hospital in Dar es Salaam which was to replace Sewa Haji Hospital dating back to the German period. Other hospital construction projects included the Mwanza area which was the most densely populated center outside Dar es Salaam. Improvements at district hospitals and the allocation of funds for hospital personnel, and last but not least for rural medical aids, would absorb the remainder of the funds under the 1956 Plan.[10] As a result, in spite of the professed continued commitment to Pridie's public health policy, the program left Tanzania's health services where they had been in 1956, with the exception of two larger improved hospitals and an embryonic program for rural health improvement.[11] In this way, an imbalance between curative and preventive health care was built into the scheme immediately before independence. The disparity was further aggravated by its dependence on territorial revenue even though its total cost was estimated at no more than 10 percent of the total revenue for the quinquiennium.[12] If the anticipated revenue should not materialize, however, allowance for its modification was made. In that case, it was stated, reduction of the rural services was anticipated.

The 1956 Plan as a whole, however, deserves favorable comment. First of all, it did not abandon preventive medicine. Furthermore, its statements on the future function of health centers point in new directions. Their role would enhance and transcend more preventive needs. They were to play a role in education and reach out to the surrounding communities in order to influence people's living conditions in their own homes. Social development was to be a part of health development. And, finally, the Medical Department was asked to set up a special health education section.[13]

In 1961, a committee was appointed by the Ministry of Health in Dar es Salaam (Titmuss Committee) to examine the existing state of the Tanzanian medical services and to suggest maximum possible improvements within a five-year period. Though critical of the slow movement of the past programs, it acknowledged their good intentions. It found, however, previous schemes lacking in one basic respect: namely, the avowed intention to provide a vast network of curative and preventive centers for the more than 8 million people in the Territory. Valuable ideas and ideals had gone into the planning of the last ten years, the report conceded, but they were not based on economic and demographic realities. Titmus and his colleagues set out to devise a more realistic program and submitted their report in 1963. But the political and economic structure of the new state underwent more changes than the Titmus committee apparently anticipated.[14] The services were not interrupted, but their growth depended in this stage on a new economic base. Before following the development of medicine in Tanganyika through the 1960s, the medical picture in Kenya must be briefly presented here.

What was observed in Tanzania also applies to Kenya. Problems of health were well defined by the 1950s. That they were not always acted on as proposed had basically the same reasons as in Tanzania. Financial restrictions, lack of manpower, investment of capital in hospitals instead of rural centers, lack of trained personnel, emergency situations during epidemics, infectious and parasitic diseases, all these factors absorbed the resources of the colonial medical budget and the subsidies of the development funds since 1945. When the director of Medical Services wrote in 1953 that the expansion of the Department had progressed steadily during the last few years, he was not wrong. In that year, however, an abrupt end to expansion came through the Mau Mau emergency.[15] To protect isolated Kikuyu peasants, they were resettled in compact villages which proved to be a successful experiment in rural public health.

Summarizing the evolution of the Kenya medical services in a 1962 report, the Ministry of Health portrayed the advance of medical development over the last sixty years as inhibited by limited financial resources throughout and always aggravated by a shortage of trained personnel. Added to that was the steady growth of the population which, again, required a continuing expansion of the services. The problems were further compounded by the ever-increasing demand for a better quality of performance. The report supported the view of the International Bank for Reconstruction and Development, which postulated health development as an investment in the productive capacity of the population, even when monetary returns were not always easy to realize.[16]

These statements sum up one of the major shortcomings of the colonial medical services. In spite of planning for growth and improvement, the services remained unbalanced. But they also indicate a change of emphasis. In the 1930s, development was made dependent on the British home economy. In 1962, it was argued that health expenses should be evaluated from the perspective of the African consumer.[17]

In what condition was the Kenya medical service when it was handed over to the new government in 1963? As elsewhere, so also in Kenya, we find in the 1950s the preponderance of curative services. The recruitment of African personnel and the setting up of rural dispensaries were recognized as almost insolvable problems. Throughout the 1950s, when it was difficult to recruit even European health inspectors for the African service, it was still more difficult to select African health assistants for dispensaries from a nonexistent pool of applicants with sufficient basic education.[18] Even when African District Councils (DCs) were made responsible for financial aid and for the selection of personnel, the problems were not solved. The ADCs employed a majority of insufficiently trained assistants and only a small number of better trained health inspectors. Even though there was some government supervision of training, the African Councils were primarily responsible for public health in rural areas. By 1957, fifty percent of ADC expenditure was funded by government but the Councils had to reimburse government for work done on their behalf. A heavy financial load was thus imposed on them and problems of quality were not solved.

In general, spokesmen for the colonial medical administration in Kenya were satisfied with attempts to expand rural health centers as a means of bringing modern medicine to the peasant population.[19] They announced with satisfaction in 1957 the addition of 25 new rural centers, which shows that they tried to update their development programs. The Kenya reports did not reflect the critical views which surfaced in 1949 in Tanganyika with the Pridie report and led to a continuing debate for almost ten years. Perhaps the closest counterpart to it can be found in the Throughton Report in Kenya in 1946. Its major theme was the indivisibility of the medical services, putting prevention and curative work on the same level. The Ministry of Health found in 1962 that it had been successful in having created an integrated medical structure which it hoped to pass on intact to the new Kenya government. It also claimed that it had "faithfully followed throughout the years" the four major points of the 1946 Throughton report, namely, the establishment of health centers, the expansion of training centers, the improvement of existing hospitals and the addition of hospital beds.[20]

When full independence was gained by the Republic of Kenya on December 12, 1963, the Ministry of Health stated that fundamental changes did not have to be made in its daily operations. But when the centralized system of government was abandoned to make room for regionalism after 1963, adjustments had to be made in the medical services.[21]

In historical perspective, it appears that the structure of colonial health administration and the extension of access to health facilities for the majority of the people in Kenya and Tanzania had been subjected to analysis and discussion during the ten years preceding independence. More and more, solutions were seen in an ever-increasing participation by Africans in the auxiliary services and to a lesser extent in the training of indigenous African doctors. The question of how to pay for hospitals and preventive care without aid from the British Treasury was left for the immediate post-war years.

6

DEVELOPMENT AND HEALTH POLICY IN TANZANIA

After independence in 1961, Tanzania's first task was the creation of a political and economic base to survive in a world of unequal partners. Decisions had to be taken on a national economy that would not have to rely exclusively on foreign investment. Geographical and ecological factors determined major choices, such as the emphasis on agriculture, the development of water resources and the struggle against disease. The leaders also focused on the social context in which to plan for economic growth. Finally, new development plans had to be drawn up at a time when the immediate course of government was untried.

The first of these plans, scheduled for three years from 1961 to 1964, illustrates the tensions of untried choices. Here was a new country that did not aim at an increase in capital formation and did not rely on a substantial rate of growth for its industry and commerce. It assigned a 24 percent growth rate to agriculture and 13.5 percent to its educational system. It set its total expenditure at £24 million, although the World Bank in a previous survey had proposed a more moderate £18 million goal. Within the total spending budget, health and labor were given only 4 percent, compared to 28 percent allotted to communications, power, and public works. These targets were not fulfilled by 1964 when the Plan ended.[1]

The second development plan extending over five years shows more planning experience. It did not depend on World Bank recommendations. It did not limit itself in its goals to the five years of the plan but anticipated changes over a longer stretch of time through 1980. The plan of 1964-69 addressed itself to the puzzling problem of why Tanzania, with 10 million people, with good natural resources and with climatic health conditions above the quality of other African countries, was nevertheless among the poorest countries of the continent. Part of the poverty was due to structural shortcomings, according to the report.[2] During the colonial period, Tanzania had to rely on primary production, and neglected manufacturing and marketing. "The economy of the country, it was said, resembled a body parts of which [had] developed normally while other parts [had] suffered from atrophy due to lack of exercize." A more ambitious program of development was therefore presented to give the country a chance to reach its full potential. One of the basic targets was an economic growth rate of 6.7 percent, although it might endanger the economic and financial equilibrium and the diversification of agricultural exports.

The social implications of the second development plan hinged largely on the rural population. The contribution of the peasantry as well as that of the more independent agricultural producers would decisively influence social changes in the rural sector and its economic productivity.[3] And it would affect health policy during the pre-Arusha period, that is, before the acceptance of socialism as the economic basis of development for Tanzania. Even though this study is primarily concerned with health and disease as an all-pervading factor in development, Tanzania's preponderantly rural population and the role it played after independence must be briefly considered here before the discussion of health schemes.

Discussions in the 1950s on the expansion of medicine to rural areas, especially in Tanzania with a peasant population of 96.4 percent, saw obstacles to cooperation stemming from a backward peasant population that was not educated and preferred to retain its customary way of life. In the 1960s, Tanzanian officials were concerned with similar problems though from a different angle. The recent literature on African communities, their role in independent national states and their ultimate dependence on a global economy has attempted to steer clear of stereotypes in explaining the farmers' resistance to change.

To get a better understanding of today's agricultural problems in Africa, historical comparisons between European peasants before and after the industrial revolution and African peasants under colonial rule will not help. The evolution of European agriculture from the sixteenth century onward is not comparable to an attempted peasant transformation under colonial administrations and since independence. During the colonial period, the peasant was faced with either producing for an international market or remaining within his limited subsistence economy. In general, he was not free to make choices like his European counterpart several centuries before, to increase his landholdings, to earn additional cash by access to new commercial centers, and the like. The colonial plantation economy, with vacillating and not always profitable exports, left the small cultivator pretty much alone as long as taxes were paid and outbreaks of epidemics, contagious disease and famine were kept under control. But it did not do much to introduce the peasant to change.

Examinations of the contemporary rural economy in Africa maintain that today's peasant producers are, with few exceptions, not better off than they were before independence.[4] Rural underdevelopment is not seen as merely the result of delayed growth due to colonial 19th century policies of keeping the periphery dependent on the metropolitan center, but rather as the product of "satellization" dating back to the 15th century and continued since. Peripheral societies are not seen as representing a stage of transition from precapitalist structures toward capitalism. They are perceived as permanent distinct capitalist formations representing a center and a periphery in the world economy.

> Underdevelopment [therefore] is not a condition of being several centuries behind the kinds of transformations experienced by the capitalist center but a condition of satellization forced upon the periphery since 1500 by the very center.[5]

From this perspective, it is difficult to see how the weakest and at the same time the largest economic group, the African peasant, can gain control of his own production and if necessary, gain support on the world market. Cliffe found that neither state-supported cooperatives, even of the ujamaa type, nor their expensive bureaucratic structure have been of benefit to the rural population in raising it above the poverty level. To properly evaluate the agricultural peasant producer's social and economic status, Cliffe suggested tracing his method of production back to the precapitalist stage and to the changes that have taken place since then.[6]

In his analysis of rural Nigeria and Tanzania, Gavin Williams defended the role which the African peasant still has to play in today's African economy.[7] He noted that African peasant producers had formerly rejected British experiments with large-scale cotton production because they did not want to lose control over their own production on their own land, which they thought fitted their needs better. British attempts to convince them of the advantages of a rational mode of production with larger crops and higher returns did not impress them. Nor did they favor colonial marketing boards. When the Tanzanian government continued similar controls after 1963, through its Agricultural Products Board acting through cooperative societies as their agents, there was similar discontent. Peasant producers were dissatisfied by what they considered as exploitation due to low prices offered them for crops which were then sold at higher prices to state agencies. Even though the government attempted to control cooperative agencies, in order to protect the peasant producer, peasants reacted at times by withholding their produce from the official market and even tried to sell in neighboring countries. Frustrated officials concluded that peasants were opposed to improvements because they were uninformed and "backward" and could therefore not comprehend why cooperative methods of production and state-controlled marketing were needed to raise their living standard and their quality of life. Noting peasant reaction, the government decided on a new approach in the 1969-74 development plan. A broader strategy was outlined to develop ujamaa villages voluntarily, using persuasion and education and avoiding coercion if possible. A 1969 presidential circular stated that, despite proclaimed socialism and despite an emphasis on the developmental rural areas, Tanzania was still a nation of peasant farmers. The ultimate objective was said to be the creation of a nation of cooperative farmers, giving them a reasonable standard of living and social benefits commensurate with the twentieth century.[8] President Nyerere described peasant productivity as most urgent in an article on "Socialism and Rural Development," saying that Tanzanian socialism must be firmly based on the land and its workers. While stressing that each person would have to produce more by harder, longer, and better work, he also referred to the importance of organized marketing and the cooperative movement in management and in its democratic machinery.[9] Williams considered the high hopes set on peasant integration into a centrally organized agricultural system as somewhat unrealistic. But he still believed in the critical role which the peasant would have to play as a class in a developing agricultural economy. He found that, contrary to appearances, peasants were quite willing to combine their efforts in the process of producing different crops. Their knowledge of local resources enabled them to adjust decisions on farm output in particular locations. They were ready to work in cooperatives if their own price demands were met without being diluted by government-imposed boards.

A recent study by Dean E. McHenry on *Tanzania's Ujamaa Villages* explains the failure of constructing a working basis for socialist agricultural production in a different way. He wrote, "the assumption that [the party] could politically socialize a diverse population in such a short time without material proof that the ujamaa village policy would significantly better village life was unrealistic." Although 90 percent of the population was resettled in villages ten years after the start of ujamaa policy, "villagization" or "living together," working together on a socialist basis, was not achieved. According to McHenry, the shift from party-directed strategy after 1967 to government-directed strategy by bureaucrats with the goal of increasing production, does not rule out the goal of ujamaa village policy at a later period. A diverse population could not be expected to accept social rural living before it had tangible evidence to convince it of the material and social advantages of such policy. He concluded that the major cause of failure was not an inherent peasant aversion to change or an inadequate educational level, but "the frequent failures of party/government officials to analyze sufficiently the nature of peasant assessment of costs and benefits to be derived from compliance."[10]

The problem connected with peasant organization, socialism, marketing boards, and world commodity prices had repercussions on the organization of medical policy in rural Tanzania in the 1960s. The rural population was faced with proposals for change from different directions. What would its reaction be to a more aggressive health policy? If its opposition to the post-Arusha medical strategy was not as outspoken as in the case of ujamaa villages, the reason may be that it had more tangible proof from the past of the advantages which modern medicine had to offer.

Planning for a comprehensive health scheme in the 1960s focused on the extension of medical facilities throughout all rural areas and was bound to link health policy closely with the state cooperative and ujamaa movement. Social and economic difficulties encountered in the peasant sector might, therefore, also be expected in the medical sphere. If the peasant cultivator was found to hold on to tradition and distrust change, he was likely not to favor changes in the existing pattern of health care. A brief survey of health policies during the 1960s and into the 1970s will examine and clarify some of these generalizations.

Just what is meant by underdevelopment of health in developing countries? Vincente Navarro introduced the question and tried to establish general criteria for this particular kind of underdevelopment. He chose as an example the Latin American country of Colombia. He found that neither the shortage of available manpower, such as doctors and medical personnel, nor the lack of a home market for health consumption were the decisive cause why large numbers of poor people lacked medical care. The real cause of medical underconsumption, he wrote in 1973, was the flow of savings and doctors from developing countries into the developed world. It drained the country, which was so badly in need of health dollars, of its financial base for health development and led to the migration of doctors. The emphasis on financing hospitals instead of spending more money on the public health sector in rural areas, did, according to Navarro, substantially damage the health of the people. Navarro's investigations led him to believe that a more equitable distribution of human resources in developing countries depended on a better distribution of their total resources which would include social and economic changes.[11]

In an examination of Tanzania's post-colonial health care, some of Navarro's assumptions do not fit the African model. In Latin America, an established upper class could direct the flow of capital investment and the importation of technology. In the African country of Tanzania, during the last colonial phase and after the assumption of national planning, consumption has not been decisively determined by a relatively small elitist group even though there existed social differentiations. The World Bank Mission was probably aware of it in its recommendations in 1960. It proposed a limited borrowing power of £11 million for 1961-1964 which would exclude heavy investment in the upper classes. The funds were to be used for roads to profit agricultural development and for education to raise the level of upper and lower-grade personnel. Though not yet officially committed to a socialist economy, Tanzanian planners based their health system on different objectives.

Nevertheless, the first three-year economic plan for 1961 to 1964 , which included the health sector, was little more than an extended budget proposal for the continuation of government services. A serious start toward a new health policy began in 1964. But as Oscar Gish has pointed out, its planners were still more representative of expatriates than of the very small number of African professionals.[12] Ideas on the role of health in Tanzanian development to 1969 were presented in an "Outline of Medical Development" by the Ministry of Health and incorporated in the first Five Year Plan. Good intentions were not lacking, broad programs were suggested, details of manpower, equipment, funds and skills were considered and detailed charts were added. The Outline was a solid piece of work. And yet, reading it at this time, after the completion of two Five Year Plans and the approaching end of the Third Plan, the 1964 outline seems to be unrealistic. One questions whether those who formulated the plan could perceive the giant task of having to propose a health model for a country whose political, social and economic structure was only just beginning to be formulated.[13] Here are some of the major points.

Medical development, it said, should produce a coordinated health service in which the Ministry of Health, local authorities and private agencies were associated. Emphasis was placed on preventive medicine and on service to rural areas; this was not merely a statement of faith but the basis of the health service. There were other basic principles also stated by colonial administrators in the preceding decades, such as the obvious postulate that health planning must aim at producing a healthy society. But one item deserves to be quoted because it was incorporated in all future plans and speeches: the healthy society was described as one which was

> free from the risks of epidemic disease, in which the individual can attain and enjoy the full physical and mental development open to him, and has a reasonable prospect of survival through childhood and normal adult years, free from the incubus of infection or preventable disorders and able to obtain medical aid when he needs it.[14]

Other general statements in the outline were so basic that they reappeared in the deliberations and programs in the succeeding years when the political and economic structure of Tanzania was changing. The test of the program, however, was the acceptance of an annual 4 percent increase in the health budget, a luxury which colonial health plans could not afford prior to the first long-range plan in 1956. The Outline further departed from previous colonial plans by its firm commitment to "a strictly limited expansion of the curative services and to use moneys thus saved for preventive medicine." It was quite emphatic in pressing the needs for health centers.

> In spite of the encouragement given by the Ministry to local authorities to establish rural health centers and especially in spite of failure of considerable financial assistance for the payment of qualified staff and the provision of equipment to persuade them to do so, the development of a country-wide system of health centers has been very disappointing. The Committee considers that the early establishment of these health centers is the most important single factor in the improvement of the health services in this country and is vital if any progress is to be made in extending the service to provide for the rural population.[15]

The cost of the plan was set at £1,600 million for capital development and £14 million for recurrent expenditure.[16]

The Plan did more than exhort, postulate, and dream about the future. It was specific, among other things, on the proposed health centers, "the most important single factor in the improvement of the health services" which should be under the direct control of the Ministry of Health until they were more firmly established. There were good reasons to fear that local authorities would lack the funds, initiative, and knowledge on how to run them. Once properly functioning, however, supervision could be shared with local authorities. Services by health centers were to include the supervision of the dispensaries, clinical care, responsibilities for the transfer of patients to hospitals, and for maternity and child welfare. They were even to serve as local headquarters for environmental operations, such as presumably malaria and schistosomiasis control and prevention. They were considered so essential that a goal of 300 was set for 1980, and 89 for 1969. But the acute doctor shortage in the 1960s precluded posting a doctor as head of the centers. Instead, health assistants were to be deputized to take charge of these vital links in the chain of an all-pervading health structure. Again, trained manpower was not yet available to staff large numbers of health centers, the key to a progressive rural medical system. The new downgraded health assistant would start without the fullest training and schooling and would, therefore, have to be placed under the general supervision of health inspectors at district headquarters.[17]

In spite of the new emphasis on health centers, hospitals were not shortchanged in the Plan for 1964-69. The old ratio of one hospital per thousand in each of the 58 districts was continued. Though ideally, hospitals below a 200-bed capacity were to be eliminated in the future, for the time being they had to be continued; where necessary, new small (and therefore expensive and inefficient) hospitals were planned. Again, as noticed many times before, the reality of manpower, funds, and material counteracted major new basic principles at every step. In part, this was due to past history. But one should not forget that the new health objectives, of country-wide rural services first advocated by Pridie in 1949 and presented from a new perspective by Titmuss in his 1964 report, were still very new and untried. Though taken seriously, they remained a goal that had to be pursued step by step.[18] In the meantime, the first Five Year Plan proposed to expand the minimum number of hospital beds to 200 within the long-term, and planned to introduce this minimum in a proportion of hospitals by 1969.

The first Five Year Plan was subjected to close scrutiny when the second Plan was drafted. The planners described medical policy during the first five years as unsatisfactory because it did not lead to a breakthrough toward a solution of Tanzania's basic health problems. It did not spread medical care vertically, from the top down to the bottom of the rural sector, where it was needed most. But it was admitted that scarcity of resources and the heavy priority placed on other sectors, such as education, resulted in "substantial neglect in the development of health services." And it was promised that the second plan would allocate more substantial resources to health development. Although by no means certain how the more substantial resources could be secured, the firm intention to allocate whatever was available made the decisive difference. In 1969, when the Second Five Year Plan was unveiled ceremoniously at a Conference of TANU, President Nyerere described the task of planning as one burdened with the greatest responsibility, that of having to make a choice. Surely, every country had problems in deciding what to choose, when and how to carry out decisions once they had been made, he said. But Tanzania's difficulty was aggravated by having to make choices between good things, not between good things and bad things. In choosing the expansion of health services, for instance, education could not be shortchanged. And in making the decision to expand rural health care, the initial poor state of hospital facilities and their serious needs could not be overlooked. But even though the First Five Year Plan had not met its goals, it was given credit for having established a basis for revamping society and the infrastructure on which it rested. Nyerere's admonition at the close of his address to TANU was dramatic and ended with the statement, "the Plan is to choose. Choose to go forward."[19] The second plan, though not too different in its objectives, was new in its strategy. It was committed to the Arusha Declaration and to a socialist form of society which medical policy was to serve and reinforce. Some of the Plan's cornerstones were not substantially different from previous ones. There was the commitment to the creation of a network of rural health centers and dispensaries which was to cover the widest possible range of rural communities. Limits were set to hospital expansion, allowing for one consulting hospital in Dar es Salaam and a limited number of regional and district hospitals in major centers of population. There was again the problem of expediting education for minimum standards of medical assistants. What was new, however, was the amount of moneys allotted for training medical auxiliary personnel and new schemes to experiment with villages, ujamaas, and state farms as centers of rural medical services.

If one compares the two Plans, a significant parallel can be detected. In 1964, the planners had to face the problem of thinking in terms of a society which was not yet clearly defined. In 1969, the Plan was based on a socialist society and economy whose operation was barely tested. Problematic situations of this kind were ominous roadblocks with which developing countries in Africa were burdened during their formative stages. Innovations and improvements had to be established on untested structures. Tanzania was aware of it. It remained to be seen how the nationalization of financial institutions, the new parastatals, and large government-controlled industries would affect spending on health and how priorities for preventive medicine would be enforced. It is not surprising that the second Plan did not reach its targets. It is more important that at the halfway stage in 1971, a re-evaluation of the Plan took place in order to readjust the goals realistically.

The growth of total government expenditure was halved when it became apparent that "the economy was under strain."[20] The health budget of 1968-69, set at TSh 19 million, was reduced to TSh 10 million in 1969-70 and projected at TSh 14 million for 1970-71. Regional planning was strengthened in the interest of rural development because it introduced interregional differentials. GDP reached 5 percent. The Ministry for Development Planning (Devplan) had improved its ability to properly assess the monetary and administrative capability of government during the Plan. More precise standards for hospital expansion, one hospital bed per 1,000 people, could be set. TSh 1,502,000 was allocated for rural health centers for 1972-73 and Tsh 50,000 was set aside for traditional medicine.[21] Did that mean that the goals of 1969 would come closer to fulfillment?

In this context, the centerpiece of the 1969 Plan,must be considered. Since rural development was seen as one of the key factors, smallscale local projects at the bottom of the pyramid by cooperative groups were preferred to minimize bureaucratic control. Crop priorities, for instance, went to cotton, tea, rice, tobacco as capital extensive programs, benefitting the largest numbers.[22]

While decentralization in rural development was seen as a prerequisite for succes, the trend was slightly different in the area of rural health. Full financial responsibility for it was returned to central government for the implementation of planning. Few rural centers had been built during the prior Plan period when recurrent financial responsibility rested with local authorities while professional supervision came from central government. Therefore, spending responsibility for all rural health centers was assumed by central government.[23] The target of 240 new rural health centers with five satellite dispensaries each for 5,000 people was now projected for the mid-1960s. But the more immediate goal of 80 new rural health centers could not be met by 1974. Even so, the government's new attitude toward rural health was called a turning point. But local authorities with little revenue found it difficult to maintain rural dispensaries even when subsidized by government.[24] It was made quite clear that basic health services, however rudimentary, must be provided *before* more sophisticated services could be increased in urban centers. On the local level, self-help construction of dispensaries was recommended. The Ministry of Health was commited to the control of funds for rural and urban centers, and it was also obligated to give professional advice together with the medical faculty in Dar es Salaam.[25]

A blueprint lends itself easily to criticism, especially when it is conceived under untested conditions. But the conception of the revised health scheme under the second Five Year Plan, with all its shortcomings, was daring in suggesting the construction of an egalitarian health system in a poor country. To better understand it, we shall try to follow the system through its critical years in the early 1970s as reflected in the observations of leading health officials, contemporary observers, and the ordinary people for whose benefit the system was set up. In this way, performances, shortcomings, wishes, and speculations may appear in a more lively perspective.

By tradition, the health budget was cast in a prescribed form, but its annual presentation to Parliament differed considerably in style and philosophy and revealed changing emphases depending on the minister who presented it. It also revealed the general climate of public opinion and specific health needs which had to be met. Each budget listed statistics on patients, on visits to the various categories of health facilities, accounts of types of disease, demographic information, and the completion or noncompletion of projects. Useful and necessary though these indicators are, they alone would not reveal the history of health and disease in Tanzania at times of social and economic transition.

The budgets of the years 1971-1976 tell an interesting story behind the facade and anonymity of officially-arrived-at data and conclusions. Most prominent in 1971 was the implementation of TANU's decision to give high priority to the development of health programs within a realistic scheme adopted for the purpose. The most important question in this context was whether there was an infrastructure on which ideologically conceived choices could be implanted together with older programs of development. Development seen as the choice between good things, as Nyerere had said in 1969, was particularly difficult in health programs because all potential choices were not only good but also needed for simultaneous implementation. In the health area, the making of choices was painful.

Another important issue in 1971 was decentralization, which was decided on because earlier programs, directed nationally, were not always enforceable on regional and local levels. There emerged, therefore, three separate health divisions, related to hospitals, manpower, and preventive services respectively. In addition, the administration wished to proceed with rural development at a faster pace, and even if it could not be done, rapid implementation of programs was demanded. No longer would it be good enough to promise paradise, but proof must be given that the government meant what it had proclaimed ever since 1969, namely, to give every citizen a chance to live without fear of disease that could be prevented by the health system. Once the issues had been stated in this way, everything reasonably possible must be done to get results.

Closely related to these issues in the health budget was the overhauling of the infrastructure. Again, the construction of rural health centers and particularly of dispensaries was to be intensified. But in recognition of the fact that the urban population—though medically better off than the rural people—must also be protected in its inalienable right to health, urban and regional hospital beds were to be increased in proportion to the growth of the population, without tilting the ratio of development toward national hospitals.[26] Figures for 1971 and 1972-73 show that the intentions were translated into action. Rural health centers increased from 90 to 97, and during the 1972-73 budget year, four more health centers were under construction and ultimately completed in 1974. The consulting hospitals in Dar es Salaam, Moshi and Mwanza on the other hand, kept their number of hospital beds at 1230.[27]

Preventive medicine was another priority, perhaps more complex because it cut across several areas. One had to discover which diseases caused major problems and why they did so. Decisions had to be made on who was to deal with epidemiology, health education, living conditions, and the cost of preventive therapy. Even when the areas were clearly defined, the borderline between prevention and clinical medicine remained muddled. In 1973, the minister of health listed malaria, tuberculosis, leprosy, sleeping sickness, measles and smallpox as the most important among forty infectious diseases.[28] Preventive medicine tied in with the hopes and expectations set on rural medicine because it might be successful in small areas where people had been alerted to self-help and an awareness of disease. But in 1974 and 1975, the health minister's speeches and WHO statements sounded pessimistic. The optimism of the years after World War II had yielded to a cautious realism expressed in a statement by the World Health Organization in 1975.

> If you happen to be born to grow up in the African bush, you are liable to have four or more disease-producing parasites simultaneously. . . . In your village every child at times suffers the paroxysms of malaria fever and your wife will mourn the death of one or two children from this disease. The snails in the village pond carry schistomosiasis. . . . If you live near a river where blackflies breed, one in ten of your friends and neighbors will be blind in the prime of life. You know that waves of killing diseases like measles and meningitis and perhaps sleeping sickness are liable to strike your village. But, lacking effective remedies, you tend to philosophize in the face of sickness. You may make an effort to walk the ten miles to the nearest dispensary when you or your child is ill, but there may be no remedies, and it may be too late.[29]

Ali Mwinyi, minister of health in 1973, advocated more extensive prevention in the battle against infectious disease and even considered preventive medicine as easily applicable. This was not the case as the accounts of the 1970s showed. WHO considered prevention of tropical infectious disease as so serious a problem in 1974 that it called for a new approach to prevention through research and through organized application of the latest available knowledge and skill, because existing methods were found inadequate to control some communicable diseases, especially the major parasitic diseases.[30] A few examples will illustrate this point. Measles, not a tropical disease and controllable in developed countries through vaccination, was still experienced as a serious problem in Tanzania in 1973, primarily for socioeconomic and financial reasons. The minister of health requested TSh 720,000 for the purchase of vaccine to raise the level of vaccination six times above its 1973 total. But vaccination alone did not solve the measles problem. It was aggravated by malnutrition. Money and education were needed to change patterns of living. Furthermore, parental ignorance facilitated exploitation by some not-so-reputable practitioners of traditional medicine who used prescriptions with no remedial impact on the disease.[31]

A greater problem was presented by malaria, in spite of advances of chemotherapy and sanitation. Malaria was responsible for 10 percent of hospital admissions and 7 percent of deaths in 1973. The outlook for the control of sleeping sickness appeared brighter in villages where education on prevention, observation of the environment, and elimination of the fly could be enforced as in ujamaa settlements. Even then, social obstacles remained a stumbling block, just as had been the case in colonial times, when resettlement of larger groups from fly-infested bush to fly-free zones had met with much resistance and little success. It was then opposed by villagers who resented interference by authorities whose orders did not make sense to them; some administrators even hesitated to use compulsion. Another disease, bilharzia, was preventable on the drawing boards, but the cost of chemotherapy and molluscicidng was prohibitive. It just was not possible to spend TSh 30 per person on bilharzia control while total per capita health expenditure in 1972 was only TSh 15. Interestingly enough, however, a year later in 1973, the cost factor was not stressed in bilharzia control. Instead, the real stumbling block was then seen in popular opposition to changing personal habits of hygiene.[32]

An evaluation of health policy of the 1970s by Minister of Health Leader Stirling in 1976 gives us a valid perspective of the complex character of the many factors involved in every decision relating to health development and thereby affecting general development policy since 1969. The minister summed up government strategy for health development under three major headings: preventive health programs, the continued expansion of rural health facilities, and the quality of hospital services. Perhaps the order in which they were listed is indicative of the emphasis placed on them. First, included in prevention were nutrition, environmental health, maternal and child health, and communicable disease. No new ideas were presented, but a continued commitment was made. Second, additional rural health facilities were pledged; and third, the quality of hospital services and technical updating was promised. The speech contained strong attacks on those who threatened the revolutionary character of the Tanzanian health system by private profit-taking, but it also appeared to coast along a previously-held moderate path toward the expansion of medical services to include all economic strata of society. It did not advocate populism versus rigid political dogmatism. Nor did it single out a shift from science toward traditionalism or the reverse. It reflected the reality of Tanzania as it was in 1976 and as such, it stressed the peculiarly Tanzanian approach to a world-wide problem within the confines of an East African political, economic, demographic, and geographic situation.

Specifically, the minister stressed an increase of dispensaries and rural medical centers depending on cooperation with the ministry of works and on the growth of training programs. The latter depended in turn on an available pool of students and on the construction of schools for training, which again could not be built as planned because of a shortage of contractors. Relief of the shortage of doctors was not expected in the immediate future, though it was urgent, with only one doctor per 23,000 in 1976. Nevertheless, the commercialization of medicine by admitting private doctors was ruled out.

> Private business of any sort [the minister said] does not accord with the policy of Tanzania, and over and above this to seek profit, to make money, out of suffering of others and especially to demand that money in the hour of trouble itself, is simply inhuman. . . . Medical aid should be a service, not a business, and here in Tanzania we are determined to bring this business to an end.[33]

But, for the time being, private units would be allowed in towns with insufficient facilities if they were run as a public service with modest fees. Charitable institutions were given similar rights.

Minister Stirling was not quite satisfied with the progress of preventive medicine, but he attributed deficiencies in the program in part to the human factor, primarily to a lack of understanding and to an unwillingness to be coerced into actions which were cumbersome, unaccustomed, and even difficult to maintain if one was asked to abandon habits like smoking or to abandon traditional preferences in food. Changes could not come overnight.

The minister of health described the major communicable diseases as the foremost targets of prevention. Although control of malaria, bilharzia, sleeping sickness, and hookworm were well-known energy wasters of the population, they continued to do harm. Prevention had become technically more difficult. The answer lay in simpler methods which the villagers themselves could apply. There was a spiral of rising prices in cloroquine for malaria patients and in insecticides for environmental control (especially against cholera). Control of tuberculosis and leprosy had reached a stage of large-scale outpatient treatment, thereby relieving hospitals. And yet the outlook was not entirely optimistic.

Again the minister appealed to all for popular participation in prevention.

> The old approach [he said] where only a few individuals were expected to solve these problems, will not carry us very far. As in the case of malaria control and the fight against malnutrition we must find new ways of collaborating among ourselves and with the people in solving these problems. For example, if people are really convinced of the harmful effects of litter, they will not stand it and may use unorthodox means to clear it, rather than wait until such a day as a spare part of a vehicle to remove the litter arrives.[34]

One can only agree wholeheartedly with the statement. The historian, however, should be more skeptical than the planners who advocated prevention. How many times in the 19th century and how many times in modern developed countries have such appeals been made without the ratio of compliance one expected. Neither police-enforced compliance nor appeal to reason have gotten rid of recurring rat problems in the slums of the most enlightened cities. This is not an objection to planning a more total involvement of everyone in sanitation.[35]

In his concluding remarks, Minister Stirling emphasized that behind statistics and scientific analyses there was the great human problem, that of the health and well-being of 15 million people being threatened by more than fifty different infectious diseases and the destructiveness of poverty.[36] The frequent references to human concerns, political necessities, underfulfillment of goals, mixed with apparent doubts regarding the prospects of coming close to the stated goals of health care for everyone in the foreseeable future, represent the present evaluation of health policy correctly. They are not a politician's cloak thrown over a web of conflicting necessities to lull the aspirations and hopes of the masses of poor peasants. They are not an indication of a lack of determination to continue to deal with health as a decisive factor in development. They stress the holistic approach to health planning and health administration because they depend on the social and economic infrastructure of a rural society which is in the process of very slow change.

This point has also been stressed by F. D. E. Mtango in an examination of the role of the doctor in rural health services in Tanzania today.[37] From his observations as an epidemiologist at the Medical Faculty of the University of Dar es Salaam, he commented on the multiple roles performed by the small number of medical practitioners of scientific medicine. Because of the national goals set for the expansion of rural medicine for the 1980s and because of the lag in auxiliary medical personnel, Mtango recommended the delegation of some of the work of the doctors to trained medical assistants. This would lessen the almost impossible task presently performed by one or two doctors in a District Hospital with responsibility for 200,000 people, with whom he could barely maintain contact. To avoid violating professional standards and medical ethics, Mtango recommended the continued upgrading of medical assistants. As he pointed out, good policies alone and a masterplan for a vast network for rural facilities in the 1980s may not be enough to cope with the facts of a rapidly growing population, the continuing increase of infective diseases such as malaria, and a continuing trend of malnutrition of 10 percent among children under five. Perhaps it is this realism which enables doctors to continue plodding ahead amidst great sacrifices toward the attainment of health for all by the year 2000, as a recent African Regional Strategy meeting proclaimed.[38]

7

RESTRUCTURING MEDICAL SERVICES IN KENYA AFTER INDEPENDENCE

In spite of differences in political organization and economic goals, the health services in Kenya and Tanzania since the early 1960s have been shaped and determined by a number of factors applicable to both countries. Kenya's medical program and problems since independence illustrate the pervasive character of medicine in eastern Africa. Disease prevention depending on financial allocations, education, training, and the acceptance of rural medicine tested a diversity of ideological assumptions and the pragmatic application of selected choices under changing circumstances.

In both countries, the colonial heritage influenced the first years of health planning in the 1960s. Kenya's prospects for economic and social transformation looked more promising in 1963 than those of Tanzania in 1961. Basically similar medical situations were approached with a different sense of urgency, and the justification of choices showed divergent views.[1] Independence came to Kenya in December 1963 after a six-month period of internal self-government. The transition from colonial medical services to an indigenous Kenyan administration was softened. The structural basis of Kenya's medical administration was strong enough to graft new plans onto it.

Both countries had comparable colonial models on which to fall back until new objectives could be formulated. In Tanganyika, the Pridie report of 1949 had debated the expansion of medical services to larger segments of the population.[2] In Kenya, a similar and yet substantially different program had been accepted in 1946. In that year, the Throughton report for Kenya's medical services had stressed the coordination of personal service, prevention, and curative medicine.[3] The report gave priority to health centers first, the expansion of training second, and an increase in hospital beds third. In 1962, the medical administrators noted with satisfaction that the report's recommendations had been followed through the years.[4] If, as the report stated, the Throughton guidelines had been faithfully observed, it represents an unusual ability to comprehend the role of medical care in Kenya. The fact, however, that in 1962 Kenya had 140 health centers and 20 subcenters whose standard was acceptable to the World Health Organization justifies the claim that the spirit of the 1946 Plan was alive. The medical services had also increased its hospital beds from 0.9 per 1000 of population in 1946 to 1.3 per 1000 in 1962, in spite of a population growth rate of 5.4 million in 1948 to 8.67 million in 1962. The existence of health centers as developed in Kenya was considered as "a major contribution to the solution of some extremely difficult problems in health service provision in less developed countries."[5] Diseases such as cholera, plague, relapsing fever, typhus, and onchocerciasis were said to have "almost vanished," although the continued existence of others was deplored. Among them were insect-borne diseases (malaria and sleeping sickness), contagious diseases (leprosy), infectious diseases (tuberculosis), and parasitic diseases. The 1962 report hoped that with the help of potent weapons like chemoprophylatic drugs, vaccines, hygiene, and education, the formidable list of as-yet unconquered diseases might be reduced. Standards had been maintained through 1962, it was said, although an expansion of the service had not taken place. This then was the situation at independence. The colonial medical administration was confident that Kenya would be able to cope with the new problems of "reconstruction to meet changing political and economic needs while yet preserving the principle of 'the indivisibility of health'."[6]

And Kenya did carry on. Immediate changes in the structure and goals of the Kenya medical system did not take place. One notices, however, the pressure of upcoming difficulties. The Ministry of Health and Housing[7] was faced with a "disappointingly large number" of resignations by the expatriate staff in 1963. In addition, local authorities faced severe financial difficulties in several areas. Changes in medical policy were coordinated with Kenya's economic development plans. The first national development plan of 1963-65 was presented to the Legislature in 1965 as *Sessional Paper no. 10* and gives many insights into the thinking of those who formulated the principles for Kenya's economic structure, its social system, and its public health policy during the formative years of the Republic.

The Sessional Paper did not present a lecture on ideology or a blueprint for future strategy. It was eclectic. There was a firm commitment to African socialism which, as Tom Mboya pointed out, accepted basic principles of socialism without enforcing dogmatism and this, according to Mboya, would permit the preservation of African (and specifically Kenyan) traditions, customs, and changing needs.[8] Kenya chose an economic policy that would be acceptable to its changing needs and would allow the selection of viable means to create economic growth as fast as possible without being bound by rigid, doctrinaire commitment. More specifically, *Sessional Paper no. 10* pledged Kenya to an economically equitable wage policy without, however, abandoning economic incentives, and a diversity of forms of ownership (state, cooperative, corporate, and individual ownership) as long as government did not lose control where necessary. Finally, planning was accepted as a means "to reorganize and Africanize the economy, provide education and welfare services, control the use of resources, etc." because, as Mboya emphatically stressed, "we must keep in mind the overwhelming need for the economy to grow."[9] The Sessional Paper and Mboya's accompanying address gave broad discretion to future policy makers with the exception of one important point: Kenya would not be bound by a Marxist ideology. The differences of future policies in Kenya and Tanzania were evident even before the Arusha Declaration of 1967.

The development of medical policy in Kenya bore out several of the principles laid down in the 1965 policy document. Recognizing Kenya's desperate need to promote economic growth in order to fulfill its goals for education and welfare, it had to overcome a vicious circle experienced by every post-colonial country in the 1960s. Mboya described it by saying "to grow faster, we must save more, but to save more we must grow faster," and therefore foreign aid and foreign capital had to be secured. Simultaneously, the goal of Africanization continued as a basic postulate. Programs in the interest of political needs at home had to contend with social and economic deficiencies such as the lack of trained administrators and insufficient numbers of professional and paraprofessional personnel in medicine. The task of bringing medical development in line with essential developmental requirements seemed enormous.

The picture which evolves from the first several years of independence is a composite of satisfaction, pride and criticism. But, whatever the shortcomings, the medical administration continued to function. Two major themes developed; one concerned manpower, and the other related to a broader distribution of medical administrative powers. The post-independence shortage of professionals in medicine followed the widespread resignations of expatriate professionals. The reorganization of government, designed to distribute powers more evenly, introduced regionalization in 1964 and a corresponding decline in quality service in many areas where the expense of rural health centers, on the other hand, could not be met by local county councils, which were still too poor to expand rural services.[10] Even if unlimited funds had been available, the replacement of doctors could not come overnight. The new Kenya constitution, aware of the burdensome bureaucracy of the colonial secretariat of the past, assigned the administration of hospitals to regional assemblies, while it reserved fiscal control to central government. This change placed regional medical officers in an awkward position. They had to deal with two masters, the provincial assembly and the central government. After one year of experimentation, in December 1964 the policy was reversed and central government resumed full responsibility for the medical services—always, however, committed to further exploration of the needs of the masses in the countryside.[11]

Free medical treatment was one of the basic rights to which Kenyans were entitled, according to the philosophy of the constitution; but, as Mboya had explained in 1965, services given by society to its people must be paid for by some one, and, in the case of Kenya, the services could not yet be entirely free. Therefore, only children and outpatients in clinics received free medical treatment as a first step. In-hospital patients had to make a contribution to reimburse the hospital. Mboya explained that it was imperative not to overburden the financial capacity of the state at this early stage of Kenya's development and growth. Individual taxation was unavoidable. He appealed to the spirit of *Harambee,* the effort of the people to help where government could not do the work at once.[12]

Looking back at the first years of health policy and its achievements, a 1971 Ministry of Health report on Kenya medicine was cautiously optimistic about progress made during the first seven years since independence; but it also pointed at social and economic factors which were largely responsible for slowing down advances. Poverty, ignorance, and a population growth rate of 3.3 per annum in

1971 were serious obstacles to the growth of public health. Among the other unfavorable factors was the continuing unemployment among the agricultural population, caused largely by arid and semi-arid areas in 80 percent of nonarable land of the territory. There were also the densely populated urban areas which created slums, disease, and poverty. The effectiveness of the teaching of disease prevention, better nutrition and family planning could not be disputed, but its impact on health and development had only just begun to make itself felt among the 90 percent of the people who lived in rural areas.[13]

To plan for an adequate health system was costly and difficult in a country whose population was unevenly distributed. In Central Province, in Nyanza, and in Nairobi, population density per square kilometer varied between 136, 180 and 790 persons respectively. In the Rift Valley in Eastern Province, it was 14, 14, and 13 per square kilometer respectively. Equally variable was the population per health center, which reached 84,000 per center in Eastern Province and 48,000 in Central Province, making it an average population of 66,000 per center, which was far too high to be effective. At the same time, per capita income was estimated at KSh 50 annually, and the rate of economic growth was given as 8.5 percent in 1970.[14] Kenya was faced with the same difficult problem that Nyerere of Tanzania had described as the planner's heartbreaking choice of selecting a few good things among the many that ought to be done. Could Kenya with a gross national budget of K£155.8 million afford to spend 6.4 percent on health, which reduced to per capita expenditure amounted to only KSh 17.50 per person?

Again, as in Tanzania, budget restrictions were a serious limiting factor, since a workable health program depended on related programs carried out concurrently. This was particularly true for rural health improvement. In 1972, the first comprehensive program for the improvement of rural health services was drawn up. It represented a departure from the more casual statements of the past because it outlined in detail the recruitment of trainees, the precise scope of their projected work, the anticipated cost, the possible delays in target dates due to related construction programs, and (perhaps the most important point) the impact of socio-economic and demographic development.[15] The 1972 proposal focused on the components of rural health as a central factor of Kenya's medical policy. By the realistic appraisal of the obstacles to performance in each area, it offered a better chance for coming to terms with the major causes of poverty, disease and ignorance.

The report chose as a target date the year 1984. The planners realized that a program as complex as rural health development must be spread out over a longer period. It would, for instance, take ten years to increase the number of medical assistants from 24 to 50 between 1972 and 1982. A competent staff for project planning would have to be secured which could not become operative until 1976.[16] Rural per capita income was not expected to grow substantially and was likely to remain at KSh 20 per annum. Recurrent budget expenses in the rural health program, on the other hand, were expected to rise from KSh 1,400,000 in 1972-73 to KSh 3,250,000 in 1984, and therefore additional funding for recurrent development spending would have to come from international sources. In the midst of all the planning for better living conditions, one expected an increase of the most prevalent and serious diseases from 10 million spells in 1972 to 16 million spells in 1984.[17] A truly gigantic task lay ahead.

The 1972 comprehensive plan for health development in rural Kenya was further implemented by detailed statistical data in 1973. The annotated and interpretive report explored the feasibility of the proposed health program under the existing financial and social conditions. It examined, among other things, the impact of demographic factors on the expansion of community health. It asked whether it was really necessary to apportion the major share of Kenya's resources to the rural sector. Statistical data seemed to support rural development. Projections showed that the rural population would increase from 9,868,783 in 1969 to 16,215,149 by 1984, whereas the urban population was estimated to increase from 1,082,000 in 1969 to 2,671,000 in 1984. There was no choice. In the light of commitments made in Kenya's Constitution, in KANU's political program, and in the philosophy of "African Socialism" as stated in *Sessional Paper no. 10,* the Ministry of Health accepted the obligation to direct an increasing share of national resources toward the rural areas.[18]

A multitude of further problems was created by the population growth factor, which was estimated to remain in excess of 3 percent per annum through the 1970s. That meant that nutritional and social services must be expanded. Money earmarked for general rural improvement, including the control of tropical disease and prevention of malnutrition, must in the future be shared with the allocation of funds for the care of mothers and infants, with family planning, and expanded education. The goal of one rural health center for every 20,000 of population was to be upheld, but growing unemployment must also be considered. The economic development of urban centers must, therefore, be matched by new sources of income for rural areas, such as the creation of small trading centers outside the major cities and towns to help the rural population economically.[19]

These considerations indicated that a strong association between socio-economic conditions and health problems was assumed by the health planners. Any projections of health planning must, therefore, reflect the significant changes likely to occur in Kenya's society in the 1970s. The interpretations of the statistical data given in 1973 are remarkably free of ideological undertones. They are pragmatic in character, relying on information relating to socio-economic trends in the past and in the future. It was stressed, however, that these trends represented only one input for health projections. An awareness of Kenya's changing productive capacity and related social adjustments in the decade of the 1970s was essential in an ongoing analysis throughout the years.[20]

The outlining of a program, however, is not enough: it must be pushed ahead to keep it alive. For this purpose, two major committees were created: one steering committee to keep the work within the confines of accepted principles, and another committee to formulate the targets. Their purpose was to prevent over-bureaucratization. Ideally, they were to maintain close contact between top planners and the lower levels of rural workers. In 1972, the formulation committee reported, for instance, on the inadequacy of rural health facilities, the shortages of staff, and the poor standards of service. The committee noted that standards could not be raised as long as people did not know how to make their homes more efficient, how to use prevention and training, especially if health workers themselves lacked the knowledge of better working performance. Primary health care required a vast educational program.

Primary health care, advocated in Kenya throughout the 1970s though not internationally formulated until 1978, is described as

> determined by social goals, such as the improvement of the quality of life and maximum health benefits to the greatest number. . . . [goals attainable] by social means, such as the acceptance of greater responsibility for health communities and individuals and their participation in attaining it.[21]

Responsibility for medical and paramedical education in Kenya was assumed by the Medical Training Center under the Ministry of Health. The Center graduated a sizable number of all types of personnel in 1978, among them 627 doctors of all categories, 885 certified clinical officers, 504 midwives, and 739 public health technicians.[22]

Kenya's third Five-Year Development Plan for 1974-1978 confirms the ideas and suggestions of the 1971 and 1972 analysis. All the previously noted economic principles, such as the coexistence of the government sector and individual enterprise, government management of major industries through the public sector, and "the greater share of production in these sectors . . . in private hands" were, at least for the time being, to continue. The goals, as earlier stated in the Second Five Year Plan of 1969, were the implementation of social justice, economic independence, an improved standard of living and particularly the promotion of rural development.[23] Specially relevant in connection with health policy during the remainder of the 1970s was the statement that,

> In spite of international economic problems we will not isolate ourselves from economic contacts with the rest of the world. . . . We shall continue to seek financial and technical assistance from friendly countries and international organizations to help us achieve the targets of the plan.[24]

The Plan gave priority to free elementary education in standard I to IV but left secondary and university training partially subsidized by individual student contributions. The range of academic training stressed the nation's need of science and mathematics during this early stage of its development. The introduction of a National Service Scheme in rural areas for students prior to their admission to the university was to involve them directly in national development and to provide a practical focus for education.[25] Even so, the danger of creating a self-perpetuating elite could not be ruled out.

As far as medical policy was concerned, the 1974-1978 Plan promised to remove as soon as possible (though within the overall constraint of national resources) the existing obstacles of inadequate resources, the shortages of manpower, and the inadequate services in the rural areas. To produce instant manpower, paramedical training was expanded and a master plan for rural medical services was to be put into effect. A new concept of health units, health teams, and family health was introduced. A health unit would serve 50,000 people, with one health center and a flexible number of dispensaries to accommodate the fluctuating growth of the population.[26] Major services, such as family planning and child health, could be performed at the health centers. To promote an acceptable and effective program of health education, local health workers were to be organized in teams under the leadership of a senior health assistant who could control and coordinate the quality of health work. To bridge the gulf between students and peasants, students were to spend one year in the National Service prior to entering a university career which, it was hoped, would give them a proper focus in educational goals related to national development. With these plans, it was assumed that the target of 161 health centers (up from 131 in 1973) could be reached in 1978. Dispensaries were to expand from 416 in 1973 to 492 in 1978.[27] "To provide useful health and family life information to 95 percent of the population" was the aim of the new system of training.[28]

The philosophy underlying the medical program of the Third Kenya Development Plan shows the influence of the most recent thinking regarding health strategy in eastern Africa and the developing world. It is too early to assess the Plan's performance. Occasional criticism in the local press and among students of public health has been directed at substandard services in some local hospitals and at the still insufficiently served rural areas in isolated regions where government-approved medical facilities have not yet been established. But these are the very reasons which have produced development programs. The displeasure with Kakamega hospital in Western Region, for instance, was disclosed by a correspondent to the *Standard* in 1976 who described it as worse than thirty years ago, with no doctor in attendance and insanitary practices which defied description.[29] Such cases prove the self-evident fact that planning for health centers, dispensaries, and training must be accompanied by the allocation of funds to build and operate the facilities that are planned.

At every stage of development, unexpected difficulties and changes in detail became necessary. In one case, the Ministry of Health adjusted the rural development program in Mbere in 1976, concentrating on operating a few important health centers instead of diffusing government effort on new units which it could not support at this particular time. Where mobile clinics had contributed to a greater demand for medical aid, the construction of new dispensaries was recommended to the Ministry of Health. Self-help efforts by local people were given credit in building dispensaries such as in Rwika, where a fast-growing population needed immediate attention.[30]

In 1978, the rural health program adopted in 1972 was substantially unchanged, although it had expanded in numbers. By then, the Ministry of Health was not only committed to the administration of rural health centers but also accepted the new concept of primary health care, described by the World Health Organization as involving, "in addition to the health sector, all related sectors and aspects of national and community development, in particular agriculture, animal husbandry, food industry, education, housing, public works, communications and other sectors," thus demanding coordinated efforts of a broad spectrum of related branches of government.[31] The concept of primary health care made health a central part of government. This trend was slow in developing, but it can be followed through three decades of health administration in eastern Africa, starting with the efforts of the colonial administration in the 1950s, through the first years of independent Kenya, and leading to a better coordinated structure in the 1970s, when health became the focus from which signals were sent out to related areas of economic and social development.

Kenya's Third Economic Development Plan upgraded the training program for rural medical assistants and recommended six rural health training centers to continue the practical training of graduates after the completion of basic training courses. By 1978, the Ministry of Health operated six of these rural medical training centers, which were run by clinical medical assistants. In three-year courses, students were instructed in medical teamwork, bringing the practice of rural medicine into line with the principles of primary health care. In fact, so basic has the idea of primary health care become for all developing countries that in 1978 an international conference meeting in Alma Ata, U.S.S.R., devoted all sessions exclusively to this subject.[32]

The Declaration of Alma Ata reaffirmed that health was a fundamental human right for all peoples of the world. It asked that the world community pledge its support to bring, by the year 2000, a level of health to everyone in order to enable a person to lead a socially and economically productive life. The key to this project was seen in the promotion of primary health care in the economically and technically disadvantaged struggling countries.

While the conference set up general guidelines for the incorporation of primary health care within the health administrations of developing countries, it listed a number of principles which were broad enough to be acceptable to governments of a variety of political regimes. In trying to cover a middle ground, its presentation of principles and the means to achieve the target of health accessible to all becomes perhaps too general to serve as a guide in the complex web of conflicting socio-economic-cultural interests of nations that differ in their geographical needs and their historical background.

Nevertheless, the Alma Ata Declaration is valuable as a model and as a guide. Its conclusions can be accepted by Marxist-oriented governments and by those with a liberal-socialist economic system. Some of the guidelines are presented here to illustrate the similarity of major health problems. The Declaration's emphasis on the interrelatedness of all sectors of development had also been stressed repeatedly in the 1974-78 Kenya Development Plan. It described primary health care as involving, for instance, "in addition to the health sector, all related sectors and aspects of national and community development, in particular agriculture, animal husbandry, food industry, education, housing, public works, communications and other sectors; and the coordinated efforts of all those sectors . . ."[33] This statement describes accurately the experience of Kenya and Tanzania in the 1970s. Even during the colonial years, the all-inclusiveness of health policy and its dependence on agriculture, education and husbandry, had been seen. The difference, however, between today's primary health care philosophy and that of earlier days is that today's postulates goals, even when the economic base barely produces a surplus to finance their achievement. Alma Ata recognizes the weight of socio-cultural and political characteristics in each country but does not subordinate them to an economy still suffering from scarcity. It postulates that money must be appropriated by directing the economy toward the objectives of primary medical care. In order for all countries to formulate strategies and national plans of action, they must be ready to exercise political will, to mobilize the country's resources, and to use available external resources rationally. The adoption of the Declaration of Alma Ata was described as "a collective expression of political will in the spirit of social equity aimed at improving health for all their peoples."[34]

This statement of principles and the commitment to affirmative action on behalf of the underserved masses of peoples in tropical, subtropical, and arid parts of the world deserves support. Equally important is the finding of human means and administrative and technological skills to carry them out.[35] Alma Ata is the logical development of earlier planning stages by individual countries which were condemned to halfway measures for historical and economic reasons. The worldwide attention which the Declaration should be given may help the struggling health strategists to continue in the right direction.

Infectious and epidemic diseases, malnutrition, the unending task of training all cadres of medical personnel, the rising birthrate, and the ever-present political problems of an East African developing country with its dependence on world economic crises are some of the factors which make the battle for health in Kenya and Tanzania a central undertaking. Health and disease in Africa are among a long list of considerations by development planners, who know that the character of their society and the stability of their industrial and agricultural structure must be supported by an economically and politically acceptable health administration.

8

TRADITIONAL MEDICINE: ITS ROLE IN EAST AFRICA TODAY

In his study of the role of the medicine man among the Zaramo in Dar es Salaam, Lloyd Swantz asked whether it was "really objective and correct to write a history of medical services in Tanzania without including the age-old and continuing practice of the medicine man."[1] In his wide-ranging study, he found much evidence of the role which the traditional healer plays today, even in close proximity to modern urban hospitals and professional practitioners of scientific medicine. In 1974, TANU gave instructions to conduct research into traditional medicine in Tanzania and to study the role which its practitioners play in Tanzanian society today, including its traditional customs and practices, in order to improve present-day health delivery.[2] In giving official recognition to this particular aspect of medicine in modern society, the Tanzanian government and the medical profession have been faced with the analysis of complex problems cutting across several disciplines. The nature of traditional healing, its pragmatic and spiritual basis, and the conditions for its coexistence with modern medicine in a developing country, have become serious objectives of study. In this chapter, therefore, traditional medicine in its colonial setting and its continuation after independence under the changing conditions of modern Kenya and Tanzania will be examined. Specifically, questions will have to be asked regarding the character of traditional healing and the value of the traditional healer among rural and urban populations. Of particular interest is the acceptance of traditionalism with its individualism in a country like Tanzania committed to socialism and state control of the professions.

Traditional medicine in abeyance: 1900-1950

The history of traditional medicine goes back far beyond the establishment of western contacts with East Africa; reading early accounts of European explorers and missionaries in Africa, however, one might easily conclude that Africans had not been overly concerned with the search for health or the control of disease. Military expeditions into the interior, away from the European fortified beachheads along the coast, and reports from missionary outposts in isolation stressed the blessing which their arrival brought to the inhabitants by introducing the rudiments of western medicine. A German army captain, not known for sentimental reflections, praised in 1903 the simple administrations of unprofessional medical aid to his African soldiers and workers as the best weapon in the conquest and pacification of unfamiliar lands. He felt that there were many people living under primitive conditions unaware of the fact that their suffering from disease required only the helping hand of modern techniques and medical treatment which their own societies had not given them.[3]

It took several decades after the establishment of British and German medical departments in East Africa before interest in African medicine and the African healer began. Discussion of the subject in the annual medical reports of the health departments were sporadic and did not show much concern, but general and professional journals reported more systematically on the use of herbs in healing and on the various types of African practitioners and their methods. Interest developed further after World War I, when European doctors made several appalling discoveries: they found that the majority of Africans recruited for service as porters in the army were physically incapacitated through malnutrition, through neglect of previous diseases, or through failure of dealing with bone fractures and their crippling aftereffects. In the 1920s, therefore, more attention was paid to the health of Africans, even if they were not directly employed on European plantations or in government camps. This change in attitude, regardless of the underlying motives, led doctors and officials to a reexamination of the ways in which Africans had reacted to health and disease before colonization and what they were doing in the 1920s. The existence of what Europeans called magic healers, sorcerers, medicine men, and diviners was not unknown to the authorities, but they did not show much interest in them as long as they did not disturb the peace.[4]

As late as 1912, at a time of a routinely established British administration in Kenya, a powerful and (according to the mission) troublesome Kikuyu headman, Kamiri, was not prosecuted for witchcraft in spite of complaints by the mission doctor, who appealed to the administration to do something about his evil magic. He described him as an official poisoner and medicine man. The British, however, preferred not to act because the alleged criminal practices could not be proven. They referred to testimony by the chief and the elders of the area, who characterized Kamiri as controlled in his behavior and always abstinent, though ill-disposed to new institutions and therefore opposed to the mission. This does not prove that British officials had a clear picture of the activities of African medicine men, but it shows that they were sufficiently puzzled by the tradition in the Kikuyu community to proceed with caution.[5] In this case, as in others that followed from time to time, the medical department–interested primarily in the good will of Africans living in the few urbanized centers–did not care to inquire into the living habits of the vast masses of the rural population. Therefore, the African traditional healer was left alone to exercise an important function of healing among his own people.

Gradually, the British administration learned to keep a fragile balance between noninterference in African customs and watchful control where and when tribal practices seemed to threaten public order. The conflict over the Kikuyu custom of female circumcision was wellknown to Kenya officials. It stemmed from the opposition to the custom by Dr. Arthur of the Church of Scotland mission in

Kikuyu and lingered on between 1909 and 1930. Opposition by the mission in Kikuyu and its board of directors in Edinburgh was justified by Dr. Arthur on medical and moral grounds. When the colonial officials were finally compelled to take a stand on prohibition of the custom or on its toleration, they decided to remain neutral as long as lives were not threatened. Prohibitive legislation on circumcision was not enacted.[6]

In Tanzania, a series of complaints about "witchdoctors" in the 1920s had led to the introduction of a witchcraft ordinance in 1929.[7] It applied only to "purported exercise of occult power" but not to the practice of the medicine man who helped good causes, such as the restoration of the affection of an estranged wife. The wording was deliberately vague because the colonial officials did not have a clear idea of the functions attributed to the traditional healer. Between 1929 and 1937, the ordinance was debated whenever a case of suspected misuse of witchcraft resulted in poisoning; very few cases, however, were taken to court under the ordinance. The colonial Secretariat in the colony and the provincial and district top officers tried to avoid sentencing suspects to prison terms or fines under the Act. It is clear that they had not made up their mind whether the traditional healer played a vital role in his community.

Several cases, reported and debated during this period at great length, throw some light on the issue. In 1933, a special cult of benevolent witchcraft called *mchapi* was observed in southern Tanzania, where it had been introduced by four men from Malawi and Mozambique in the border district. The men held meetings for the entire population of the towns they visited, swindled the population out of considerable sums of money, and disturbed their peace of mind. Their methods were described as intentionally fraudulent. They also sold a medicine called *mchapi,* which was given as protection against present and future evil magic and served as general medicine against natural diseases. In this case, the government took action and deported the men across the border into Portuguese territory.[8]

Why were British officials so hesitant to take action? In opposing criminal prosecution in almost every case that came up between 1929 and 1937, Provincial Commissioner A. E. Kitching made several points. Only black art (*uchawi*) was criminal. It must be distinguished from *uganga,* the diagnosis and treatment of disease, including witchcraft. *Uchawi* had evil intentions; *uganga* could be described as "a science, practiced no doubt by many charlatans and not always with benign intentions but nonetheless a science."[9] He was convinced that the serious character of an honest traditional healer-waganga could be distinguished from the cheating and dishonest manipulations of a crook, but he questioned the value of an amended witchcraft ordinance which was not intended as a serious piece of social legislation. It would not assist, he thought, in any way "towards the eradication of the beliefs and fears which haunt and obsess the minds of natives and oppress their lives as nothing else does. . . ." "*Uchawi,*" he wrote, "was not a noxious weed to be pulled up by the roots or sprayed with arsenic but the greatest social problem confronting native administration."[10] We may conclude that Kitching was not concerned with the threat that *mchapi* presented to European medicine. Two Christian missions in the area, the Benedictines and U.M.C.A., were absolutely opposed to *mchapi.* Mohamedans also took a stand against it. The government maintained its aloofness, as long as it hoped to achieve through education what imprisonment and fines would not do: namely, an awareness that the traditional healer could do less than modern scientific medicine.

The traditional healer did not change his methods and concepts substantially after he came into contact with western medicine during the decades of coexistence with Europeans in the twentieth century, but the non-African world has come to a deeper understanding of African medicines and primitive societies in the course of their extended contacts since World War I. Especially during the last twenty years of the colonial period and since then, anthropologists, sociologists, medical experts, and recently also historians, have analyzed the nature of traditional medicine, the character of the traditional healer, and the concepts on which they based their action.[11] It is appropriate to give a few generally accepted explanations of the medical, socio-religious, and cultural concepts on which traditional and religious men based their art of healing.

Concepts and practices of traditional medicine

The western outsider trying to comprehend the system of African traditional healing was confounded by the conflicting terms used by native societies for their medicine men. They saw East African traditional medicine, like primitive medicine in earlier societies, rooted in a world of magic dominated by supernatural forces at the same time it responded to natural causes of disease which could be detected by rational observation. This unique toleration of the coexistence of heterogeneous factors seemed incomprehensible to the scientifically trained observers of the African scene, so much so that they questioned the value of a system that used magic and the advocacy of spirits together with the dispensing of herbs whose effectiveness could be objectively tested.

Erwin Ackerknecht described the conflicting elements of traditional medicine in a clear and precise statement that is quoted here to set the scene for our discussion of traditional medicine. After noting that the treatment of disease in primitive societies was not exclusively magico-religious, but that it accepted methods of rational treatment, he continued, "As far as the proportions between rational and supernaturalistic concepts and methods are concerned, it seems that *primitive medicine is primarily magico-religious, utilizing a few rational elements, while our medicine is predominantly rational and scientific, employing a few magic elements.*"[12] The overpowering existence of belief in a world ruled by magic forces was mitigated by the diviner, who had the ability to interpret the magic roots of illness and misfortune to the innocent victims of pain and suffering.

The apparent contradiction implied in the use of rational observation in determining the natural cause of certain more easily explainable diseases and the use of spiritual divination in explaining the more complex causes of imbalances in sick persons can only be comprehended if one examines the total universe as the traditional African sees it. Ackerknecht made it clear that causality in our sense does not exist "in a magical world where the natural is supernatural but the supernatural quite natural."[13] An African Assistant Secretary in the office of the British colonial Medical Services in Tanzania, when asked to write a memorandum on African Medicine in 1933, found it quite difficult to reconcile the contradictions between

African religious concepts and the African medical concepts of the healer. He gave a brief presentation of African religious concepts which he described as so interwoven with the African laws, customs, and medicines, that it was almost impossible to separate one from the other. "The whole movement of the primitive African [he explained] from morning to evening until the time he goes to bed is guided by his religious tenets. He so strictly observes them that he hardly moves about without referring to them for guidance, and this is why an African is by nature superstitious."[14] In describing the pervasive character of African religious beliefs, he hoped to make the modern scientist comprehend why a diviner, i.e., a religious man, with a special gift of conversing with supernatural forces, was the major source in determining and prescribing a cure for an illness. Once the cause had been found, the application of the herbal medicine was left in the hands of a herbalist if a "natural" cure was proposed. The major part of his memorandum detailed the medicines used by the herbalist rather than witchcraft used by the diviner.[15]

Some thirty years later, John S. Mbiti, at the time professor of theology at Makerere College in Uganda, gave a detailed and scholarly description of the world of spirits which has played a leading and vital role in much of everyday African life and has shaped African attitudes toward health and disease.[16] Although the number of spirits, their functions, and their role in the nonmaterial world varies according to different tribes and different geographical areas, Mbiti found conceptual similarities broad enough to set forth several general characteristics. They are helpful in trying to give meaning to the term "magic" used so indiscriminately in many accounts of African medicine. He noted the following criteria.[17] First, the presence of spirits, i.e., nonmaterial beings who play an active role in peoples' daily lives, in their moral aspirations and in their general social behavior, represents a reality for the traditional African. It determines his attitude toward health and disease. Second, within the hierarchy of beings in the nonmaterial world, spirits occupy an intermediate position below the "divinities" and above the "living-dead." Third, the divinities represent primarily God's activities and manifestations and, with the Ashanti, God even manifests Himself through them. Finally, beneath the divinities, there are the spirits which though invisible can make themselves visible to human beings under certain conditions. As a collective group they were thought to have immortality, and though they were feared by humans who did not know their intentions, they were not considered to be either good or bad as such. Their dwelling places have variously been described as underground, in woods, bush, forests, and rivers; most likely they reflected the living conditions of those who assigned geographical areas to them. Generally, the spirit world is conceived as invisible and differs from the human world. It creates a feeling of security as well as insecurity at the same time, something that early non-African observers interpreted with skepticism when speaking of "beliefs and fears which haunt and obsess the minds of the natives and oppress their lives."[18]

The spirits were described as intermediaries between God and the living world. However, the living-dead, a group of spirits below the true spirits, were most likely seen as intermediaries between the spiritual world and the world of the living human beings, since they had once been alive and were familiar with the needs of the human beings in their physical surroundings. Mbiti suggested that they were welcome to their former quarters when they appeared, but that a prolonged stay was not wanted. Or, as he stated it, "the living-dead are wanted and not wanted."[19] One was never sure whether they watched over the wellbeing of their clan and their country.

What influence did these religious concepts have on people who lived in tropical regions open to attack by insects, wild animals, natural catastrophies such as sand-storms, crop losses, floods, migrations from other zones and, in certain areas, in nearly total isolation? Their need for protection made the world of magic almost a postulate and created a dual attitude toward protection from disease. In this world, the diviner who conversed with the spirits became the major consultant when disease struck.

The diviner's role in past and present African life follows logically from the African concept of religion, yet this role was mystified and misrepresented by westerners after they established contact in Africa in the latter part of the nine-teenth century. There are a number of explanations for this confusion. Belief in a world populated by spirits made survival in the physical world largely dependent on the relations between human beings and their spirits. Ill health, misfortune, and social frictions which defied simple and plausible explanations, were attributed to supernatural causes. The diviner, who was credited with the ability to respond to the spirits responsible for family and community, was the authority to decide what went wrong and what caused a particular illness, pain, or bad luck.

In most descriptions of the diviner in African society, it is the diviner who detects the cause of disease and follows up with his treatment on the basis of supernaturalistic premises and with the aid of herbal medicine. But contrary to the western doctor who takes his patient's medical history, the first concern of the diviner, as Lloyd Swantz has shown, is not *what* caused a particular disease but *who* caused the illness that befell the sick man and how the patient can be protected in the future from becoming again the victim of evil forces.[20] After that question has been answered, the patient may be treated by magic and herbal medicine dispensed by the diviner, or he may seek the help of a herbalist who does not do any divining, or he may even seek help from a modern hospital. The diviner's task is primarily to locate the dissatisfied ancestor or the force that put the spell on him or the member of his own community that tried to bewitch him. The diviner has been described by various tribes as a wise man, a benefactor, a seer. But he antagonized those whom he accused of being responsible for illness, lack of rain, epidemics, and all kinds of misfortune. The person so accused might turn against the diviner and call him a sorcerer.[21] This led to a confusion of terms and made the magic healer appear in many different functions which were not always understood by early traders, explorers, missionaries, and even anthropologists, who might often learn of his work only by hearsay. The image of a diviner or magic healer could easily be mistaken as that of a charlatan or superstitious im-poster, although no one denied that charlatans were among the diviners. Recent analyses have attempted to tabulate the diviner's activity more objectively.

C. K. Omari tried to classify the terminology on the traditional healer by dis-tinguishing between ethnicity, the terms used by ethnic groups, and the character-istics which these groups assigned to the healer.[22] The striking thing is that the *mganga* (Swahili for healer) is described by four ethnic groups most frequently as wise man, diviner, seer, curer, protector, healer, rainmaker, and a man who performs good acts and is harmless.

Although all African tribes believed in supernatural causation of disease, the ratio between supernatural and natural causation varied according to ethnic groups. E. E. Evans-Pritchard tells us that the Azande attributed nearly all sickness, whatever the nature, to witchcraft or sorcery, and that in order to cure a serious illness, these forces must be defeated. He added, however, that Azande did not entirely "disregard secondary causes, but in so far as they recognize these, they generally think of them as associated with witchcraft and magic."[23]

Accepting magic and natural causes of disease, the task of the healer is largely removed from the rational, although we shall see later that a number of East African healers had elaborate lists of plants and the specific uses to which they could be put.[24] To have a broad basis for our discussion of traditional medicine in Africa today, the definition given by a committee of experts in 1976 at their meeting in Brazzaville may serve as a basis for further analysis in this chapter. According to the report,

> traditional medicine might . . . be defined as the sum total of all the knowledge and practices, whether explicable or not, used in diagnosis, prevention and elimination of physical, mental or social imbalance and relying exclusively on practical experience and observation handed down from generation to generation whether verbally or in writing.[25]

In their discussion of traditional medicine, the experts stressed its nonscientific character, emphasizing the nature of the basic ideas underlying it. Traditional medicine did not regard man as a purely physical entity but also took into consideration the sociological environment, whether living or dead (ancestors), and the "intangible forces" of the Universe (spirits and gods).[26]

Traditional medicine in East Africa survived the colonial period. In fact, it developed and in some instances made adjustments to western medicine. Diviners and healers did not object when their patients consulted government doctors or went to hospitals, as long as they had at least been diagnosed by their own healers. Articles written by medical officials, administrators, and mission personnel between 1930 and 1950 confirm the coexistence of the two systems and the greater interest which both sides took in each other.[27] Traditional medicine, though not recognized as part of the medical system in East Africa, was given consideration as a significant aspect of African rural life. Officially, the medical departments of Kenya and Tanzania maintained their attitude of aloofness toward the traditional healers or *mganga.* Between 1946 and 1953, witchcraft cases were brought to the attention of the Colonial Secretariat from time to time. They were investigated after reports had been received about planned acts of sorcery and were routinely dismissed.[28]

But traditional medicine was not considered as a subsidy to supplement the paucity of medical services in rural areas. On the contrary, when an increase of medical helpers and rural dispensaries was debated in Tanzania in 1955, it was also done with an eye to counteracting the native system of medicine through magic. Exorcism, for instance, aroused the suspicion of authorities, although it was part of *uganga* (benevolent medicine). It was used as a means of driving out evil spells by witches or sorcerers who might destroy the community. The ceremony used in exorcism might impress the non-African observer as irrational cultism and, therefore, meaningless to the scientific observer who practiced medicine.[29]

Apart from the official attitude toward the traditional healer during the final years of colonial government, one finds a good deal of literature for the period written by interested observers. It gives us a more balanced evaluation of how the outside world perceived the *mganga* (traditional healer). In a study on the Digo of East Africa, L. P. Gerlach concerned himself with the contradiction of logical conclusions and magic in his presentation of Digo conceptions of health and disease.[30] Diagnosis, he wrote, proceeded in a logical manner, but it was based on the unscientific Digo premises as to the cause and effect of illness. The fact that logical conclusions were drawn from nonlogical and nonverifiable assumptions caused many misinterpretations of the relationship between magic and natural treatment in traditional medicine. The average Digo would first determine whether illness was natural or God-sent and treat it with herbs, roots, or patent medicine available in stores. If improvement did not come, he would consult the *mganga* to discover what taboo had been broken, what particular treatment was required, whether sorcery was the cause. This would be followed by rituals, chanting, and trance, until the name of the spirit or the member of the community responsible for the illness was revealed. One finds a combination of first searching for a logical explanation and then resorting to supernatural revelation. Similar descriptions can be found for many parts of East Africa.

The writer of the aforementioned essay on "African Medicines," who interpreted African attitudes toward disease to the British administration in 1933, added to his long list of herbal remedies a section on diseases which the African treated through exorcism of the devils, which were believed to inflict certain diseases. In such cases, the diviner recommended specific doctors capable of appeasing the client and his family and of relieving him of the suffering. This was done at ceremonial gatherings of the family or clan, called the big *ngoma,* at which the patient danced until in entrancement he was able to name the devil responsible for his illness. If the guilty party was not located, the victim was ordered to join the devil dancers for the rest of his life. This kind of treatment for exorcism was expensive, time consuming, and did not always lead to a cure.

Other methods of treatment mentioned by this writer were herbal medicines, root medicines, bark medicines, incisions, cupping, amulets, treatment of snakebite, bleeding, leprosy, fever, and constipation. He concluded his report by saying, "it will therefore be seen that Africans have got medicines for various diseases, some or the majority of them I have not mentioned here." No distinction was made by him between natural prescriptions and the use of magic and ritual.[31]

Although Africans distinguished between white and black magic, the transition was often without clearcut differentiation, and the community might not be able to draw the line between legitimate and criminal uses of witchcraft accusations. On the whole, unsubstantiated witchcraft accusations were kept to a minimum to avoid the high cost of ritual defence.[32] One factor emerges, however, from the early descriptions of white and black magic. As Robert Gillan from the Church of

Scotland Mission at Tumu Tumu explained in 1930, white magic practiced by a medicine man (*mundo mugo*) was beneficial to the person it claimed to protect. It might consist of medicine like calabash tips or tips from goats' horn around the body as a preventative device against disease, but it was not envisaged as having immediate healing properties. White magic was also used to trace the cause of loss or suffering inflicted by a witch or a demon. Blacksmiths and bewitchers (*arogi*) were identified with black magic, which was dreaded more than anything else because it was shrouded in secrecy. It could be carried out from a distance, at the blacksmith's place of work. Spells could be cast on nonsuspecting persons. Gillan found that the practitioners of black magic were often described as persons with unfavorable physical characteristics, misanthropes, social rejects who wanted to settle a grudge–in other words, persons with a negative attitude toward their community.[33]

This observation is borne out by a much later report on black magic in 1953. In this case, a young man with no apparent cause for resentment was accused of responsibility for two consecutive seasons of hailstorms and ruined crops. His image in the community was a negative one, probably because he was a newcomer who had lived there only for two years. He was a landless peasant from another tribe who found himself rejected. He then threatened to destroy peasant crops by unloosing hailstorms, which he said he could order at will. The unusual arrival of hailstorms shortly thereafter incensed the peasants so much that they dragged the man to the District Officer. When he testified under oath that he had no power to send hailstorms, a power which only God could exercise and that the people were telling lies, the District Officer found him guilty of another offense. He was accused of falsely boasting of having the power to produce hailstorms and of having caused unrest among the villagers. He was temporarily banned to live in another area.[34]

The literature on the medicinal value of herbal remedies and the methodology of their application prior to 1960 has been widely reported. It was in this area that foreign observers trod on firmer ground and were more specific in their observations. Only a few examples are selected here to give an idea of the great variety of plants, roots, and bark used by healers against a number of diseases. The title of an article published by Dr. Weck in 1908, when he was staff-surgeon in the German protective force (*Schutztruppe*) in East Africa,[35] reveals his respect for African traditional medicine. He wrote on "The Wahehe Doctor and His Science" at a time when African healers were hardly taken seriously. These doctors, he wrote, were not merely practicing magic. Their concern was the healing of the sick, a profession known among the Wahehe throughout their history before the arrival of the Germans. He mentioned that the practice of medicine was open to both men and women. Specialists for specific diseases did not exist. The Wahehe healers were particularly knowledgeable in general medicine, but they seldom performed surgery, an observation made also by other writers on African medicine. Before treating a person, they examined his body with their hands without using an instrument, as Dr. Weck specifically stated. Primarily, however, they were concerned with the selection of the correct medicine for the particular disease they diagnosed. As for surgery, they had learned suturing from the Arabs in East Africa, but they seldom applied it. Dr. Weck was impressed by the level of Wahehe traditional healing. To substantiate his report, he added a list of more than fifty diseases and their pathological symptoms, which he found correct in the majority of cases.

This early report, written before World War I, was confirmed by others in the years following the war. W. D. Raymond, government chemist in Dar es Salaam, wrote a series of three articles on *materia medica* between 1936 and 1938.[36] He described arrow poisons, some of which killed monkeys instantly and antelopes within minutes. Among the drugs and powders used by Africans in Tanzania during his time, he found the drugs made of herbs quite effective in many diseases, whereas the powders were relatively ineffective except for illnesses attributed to witchcraft. Altogether, Raymond listed twenty-seven medicinal plants. Among the list of medical and poisonous plants cited by Hans Cory were roots used for sexual stimulation, tapeworm treatment, and others.[37] Raymond's research showed that the danger of infectious disease was wellknown, but as Dr. Weck had noted earlier, the transmission of malaria through the mosquito was either not known or not accepted.

By the end of the colonial period, traditional medicine, though still primarily seen in its magic context, was recognized by Europeans as a profession of specialists. It was an aspect of African life that had not been eliminated by the building of roads, ports, railways and a few cities in Kenya and Tanzania. Even dispensaries operated in the bush by young African helpers, who dispensed aspirin and anti-malaria drugs, coexisted with the traditional healer. In 1933, the Chief Secretary of Government in Dar es Salaam decided to leave the registration of the native doctor to a later period when more would be known about him and his ability to cooperate with the established medical system.[38] In 1939, Lord Hailey suggested in his *African Survey* that more attention be paid to the study of herbs used by practitioners of native medicine in order to incorporate them into a list of medicines used by western doctors. In the same year, the Conference of Directors of Medical Services, meeting in Nairobi, expressed themselves in agreement with Lord Hailey and confirmed that the study of native medicines had been included in the East African research program.[39] After 1960, the role of traditional medicine would have to be reconsidered. Would it be able to cope with the changes in political and social organization in Kenya and Tanzania?

Traditional medicine in spite of development: the years of transition

When the medical departments assessed their status after independence, they did not mention traditional medicine. One must assume that its continuation, side by side with modern scientific medicine but apart from it, was taken for granted and was not considered a special issue.

In Tanzania, the problem of raising productivity and the standard of living of the rural sector (which contained 96 percent of the population) had first priority in planning for the years immediately following independence. With it went the pledge to give priority to preventive medicine, and, for that reason, to expand dispensaries in order to have a countrywide system of health centers. Eighty-nine rural dispensaries were planned for 1969.[40] These objectives lent themselves to a continuation of the policy of benevolent neglect or tolerance of rural healers.

There were other considerations, too. Since there was no official policy on traditional medicine, conclusions regarding this period can be drawn only from the scarce material available in articles written during the early years after 1960. There were some basic questions which had to be considered sooner or later. Tanzania, for instance, was held together by a mass party, TANU, which had only been founded in 1954 and had very little time to consolidate its ideas before independence. Tribal allegiance could not be discarded overnight as a factor in nation-building. The goal of African socialism was more of an ideal than a structural base serving as the only formative and uniting factor in national unity.

Against this background, traditional medicine—with its belief in a nonmaterial culture based on religion—was an untested force in the search for ideological unity. Omari made this point clearly when he wrote, "to understand people's culture before setting up some machinery of implementing a policy or setting up a programme for development of the people is as important as knowing the ecology of the area."[41]

Scientific medicine was considered vital in developing Tanzanian society, just as technological improvements were. Was there a danger that traditional medicine might weaken the determination to train as many young doctors as possible during the two development plans between 1961 and 1969? And even if the scientific training of doctors, paramedical help, and rural medical auxiliaries, was upheld and adhered to, would the peasants in remoter villages be ready to accept them as long as traditional healers were nearby?

Among those who were in touch with traditional healers in Tanzania soon after independence was Dr. P. I. Imperato, who spent some time in North Mara district with the Luo in 1961-62. He was aware that his observations on "Witchcraft and Traditional Medicine Among the Luo of Tanzania" were collected at a time of political change and might be considered merely of historical value.[42] But later reports by other writers in the 1970s show that his statements maintained their validity. He observed that even an educated person in a village could hardly disregard tradition, mainly because "the overwhelming and comfortable routine of rituals conveyed the authority and assurance which often stem from age and experience."[43] Imperato found that the Luo believed in three kinds of evil witches and sorcerers. They were thought to attack the "psychical parts of the victims' organs." Repeated attacks might kill the victim. The safest weapon against attacks by witches might be for a person to leave the village. Equally dangerous were the sorcerers. They might harm persons by slipping poisons containing strychnine into the victim's food or drink. But the greatest danger was presented by the combination of witchcraft and sorcery in the person of the witch-sorcerer (*jajuok*), who could destroy entire families and villages. Fortunately for the Luo, they also had good witch doctors who could use countermagic to protect the community. But believing in evil witches and sorcerers as the Luo did must have presented an extremely threatening social atmosphere.

Imperato's observations on Luo concepts of disease and on doctor-patient relations are not dissimilar from descriptions of traditional medicine during the colonial period.[44] The Luo concept of disease was not based exclusively on magic.

They may have experimented with different medicines and attempted to relate symptoms of disease to physical causes. But generally their attitude toward disease was unscientific. For example, they did not attribute anthrax to cattle, but rather to drinking dirty water or to eating the wrong combination of food. They did not observe or suspect a connection between trypanosomiasis and poaching game along the fringes of the Serengeti Plains. For years, medical officials had had similar problems when they tried to enforce the separation of men and cattle from tsetse fly in their attempt to prevent the spread of trypanosomiasis. Imperato also noted that the Luos' knowledge of anatomy was limited, and surgical treatment was done only by a small group of specialists. This may explain their inability to trace certain diseases to the correct anatomical parts of the body. Yet, like many other African tribes, they were able to treat major diseases like onchocerciasis, pulmonary ailments, and syphilis with herbal prescriptions. The influence of the traditional healer on the Luo community was significant. Practitioners of western medicine might find themselves suddenly deserted by their patient when he decided to seek help from an African healer. Often patients tried to combine western treatment with that of their own healer, and there were others who would not consult a western doctor at all. This pattern of behavior can still be observed in East African hospitals to this day. Similar observations with slightly different conclusions were made by Dr. K. Ndeti in an article on the relevance of the African traditional doctor in scientific medicine. His examples referred mostly to the 1960s.[45] His observations are particularly valuable because he was trained in scientific medicine and, at the time of writing, was a member of the Community Health Department of the University of Nairobi.

In his paper, he addressed an academic audience of scientists whose skeptical attitude he seems to have presumed. With great objectivity, he first described the accusations made against the witch doctor. He mentioned the aura of mystery that accompanies his diagnoses and therapies, his lack of scientific training, his ignorance of scientific theories (germ theory, for instance), and his interpretation of cause and effect in the course of disease. Instead of concentrating on the scientifically ascertainable facts of diseases like gonorrhea, syphilis, schistosomiasis, and others, he relies on spirits of ancestors and their role in causing these illnesses. But then Ndeti retraced his steps and gave examples of the traditional healer as the wise man with a noble outlook, who took his work seriously and prepared himself for his trade. He described specific cases of patients who had left western treatment because they did not regain their health in a western hospital or with a private practitioner of western medicine, but who were healed when they transferred to the traditional doctor.

Even though he gave full credit to antibiotics, the skills of modern surgery, the sophistication of the modern doctor and "other landmarks in the stride of modern medicine," he maintained that the traditional doctor has a role in our modern system of medicine. His arguments were much more provocative ten years ago than they are today, at a time when the humanistic approach to medicine and an emphasis on the doctor-patient relationship are stressed. He saw the importance of the interplay of physical body and the cultural-social environment. Especially in view of the vital importance of preventive medicine in East Africa's medical climate,

Ndeti's plea for more serious consideration of native behavioral reaction to disease control and disease prevention makes sense. Ndeti listed the effectiveness of the traditional doctor in three areas. He gave him credit for (1) the treatment of specific diseases with herbs, (2) the herbal treatment of symptomatic diseases with a psychological result, and (3) the treatment of psychological diseases through psychological therapy.[46] He did not ask for the abandonment of scientific progress but rather for acceptance of the reality of the traditional healer "as a very important part" of modern society with a "legitimate knowledge essential for medical science."[47]

Dr. Ndeti's acceptance of the native doctor as part of the social and cultural structure in East Africa in the 1960s must not be confused with the genuine rejection of and even repugnance to the witch doctor whose purpose was destruction or death. An interesting example was cited by the leading Uganda newspaper in 1964. It told the story of 200 witch doctors who surrendered voluntarily before a crowd of 3,000 people at Baricho, Kirinyaga district. A leading member of the group of witch doctors apologized publicly for having bewitched and caused the death of nine men and women from his own clan and promised to abandon witchcraft for good. The surrender took place in the presence of members of Uganda's Parliament.[48]

Gradually, the benevolent neglect that had characterized the relations between scientific and traditional medicine for several decades began to yield to an attitude of benevolent curiosity. Western doctors and native African doctors began to study the differences in concepts and patient treatment of the two systems to establish areas of cooperation. Mark T. Bura,[49] for instance, investigated Wairaqu concepts of diagnosis and treatment of disease. He established data on the Wairaqu, a tribe of some 180,000 in the Arusha region, by questioning them directly. He wanted to know more about their method of diagnosis, the treatment recommended for diseases, and the measures recommended to prevent disease. His tabulation shows that only diseases with minor complaints were self-diagnosed, among them the common cold, mild headache, fever, chronic abdominal pain attributed to food, superficial malignancies, and fractures. The majority of symptoms was submitted to a diviner for diagnosis. From the diseases listed in this category, it appears that unusual complaints or symptoms without an obvious cause were referred to the diviner. In these cases, one may infer that the fear of the unknown and unpredictable source of the illness convinced the sick person of the supernatural origin of his complaints. In this situation, only a diviner, acquainted with the spiritual world, was trusted witht the dispensing of medicine aimed at the spiritual world. Bura recommended that the medical worker study the tribal medical system in order to understand why the medical services offered by government were often not fully appreciated and where they had failed.[50]

Another approach was carried out by two doctors who attended sessions between a diviner and his patient. I. G. A. J. Hautvast and M. L. J. Hautvast-Mertens studied such a session in a Nyakyusa (Bantu) community. Since traditional Bantu medicine attributes most illnesses to witchcraft, the authors reported the session verbatim to make western-trained practitioners aware of the depth of Bantu beliefs among the people they treated with their advanced modern techniques of diagnosis without fathoming the gulf that separates them culturally and therefore affects the conceptual framework of disease.[51] In the case which they reported, a woman consulted a diviner to find out why her adult son was sick and whether and how he could be cured. The discussion between the woman, the diviner, and the two spirits summoned to the session was a nonrational reconstruction by the diviner, with the aid of the spirits, to determine a plausible cause of the ailment. The diviner reported to the woman that a piece of sugarcane given to her son by a person bent on his destruction remained in his body and could be removed with the help of a traditional doctor. In this way, the woman was assured that the son could be restored to health by a medicine man, and in this case did not have to go to a hospital.[52] The authors identified a number of diseases which the Nyakusa interpreted as sent by God and natural in origin, diseases which did not require spirit intervention. They listed other diseases as caused by spirits, magico-religious in origin, and solvable only with the aid of the traditional doctor. They concluded, on the basis of evidence, that as long as belief in witchcraft continues to exist among the Bantu, "one has to realize, for the time being, that it will exist side by side with the modern western pattern." The mode of interaction of the two systems remains an open question.[53]

Traditional medicine after the Arusha Declaration

Major political changes in Tanzania after 1965 influenced the selection of new targets for health in the Second Five Year Plan in 1969. Commitment to the post-Arusha strategy with emphasis on equality, self-reliance and democracy[54] meant in terms of health that government must mobilize all the resources of the country toward the elimination of poverty, ignorance and disease.[55] In general terms, this included everyone's right to protection, regardless of his ability to pay or his place of residence, close to or far from medical facilities. The post-Arusha policy also included the commitment to socialist agricultural villages (*ujamaa*), which required education for future communal living in villages. The trend toward villagization, though it did not reach the expected goal of the *ujamaa* type socialist settlements,[56] introduced a new element in the style of peasant traditions. Would the traditional healer, steeped in a philosophy of individualism, with attachment to clan and family, be left out of the new program?

The traditional healer, as a diviner and as a herbalist, had been on his own, aloof from government control under normal conditions. This had been one of the major objections. His secrecy made the medical profession and government uneasy. When the new agricultural program required TANU supervision in the villages, it appeared questionable whether traditional healing could continue as before, but the opposite happened: traditional healing proceeded in a new direction. A new trend toward coexistence, with the approval of the state and the medical profession, began in the early 1970s.

Five major reasons brought about the reversal from polite toleration and benevolent neglect to a strategy of planned integration. *First,* an awareness of the value of traditional medicine was expressed at regional meetings throughout Africa. The meetings were assisted by WHO, though not officially endorsed by the World Health Organization. *Second,* an ever-growing shortage of resources and manpower essential for the continued expansion of all types of curative and preventive services in all African states had been reported. This referred in particular to Tanzania, with its goal of a vast scheme for rural health development. *Third,* even urban centers have increasingly experienced the continuing practice of traditional healing, although it appears to be inconsistent with the rapid changes toward modernization in cities. *Fourth,* since 1974, TANU has been instrumental in promoting research into traditional medicine and its ramifications. *Fifth,* a world-wide skepticism regarding the extreme application of technology to medicine and the underutilization of the human factor in medicine has facilitated the African approach to the once almost-discarded practice of traditional medicine.[57]

Although the interest in traditional medicine is Africa-wide, Tanzania is chosen in this section as an illustration of the latest developments. It has established an organization to investigate the problems of coexistence, and it is on the way to taking administrative and legal steps in that direction. It gives us, therefore, an example of a more realistic appraisal of the role of traditional medicine in Africa today. When TANU took an interest in research in traditional medicine in 1974, it concentrated first on the use of herbalists to supplement its supply of medicinal drugs with the medicinal plants available in Tanzania. It is this aspect of traditional medicine that lends itself most readily to cooperation with scientists, i.e., chemists, microbiologists, immunologists, botanists. In 1978, a list of sixty-two Chinese medicinal plants that grow in Tanzania was prepared by Dr. Madati, Chief Government Chemist, together with a list of their active principles.[58] The ever-increasing cost of drugs and the growing skepticism of their potential damage to health, in spite of the perfection of their production based on research, has created an atmosphere in which the medical use of herbs is being examined. Since, as Madati showed, only TSh 6 per person is available for health in Tanzania, not more than TSh 2 can be expended on imported drugs, which is not enough in a country with malaria, tuberculosis, schistomiasis, trypanosomiasis, and other diseases which require large amounts of drugs. In spite of his advocacy of the use of the "natural" constituents of the drugs, Madati is aware of the danger of their toxic ingredients and recommended their expanded use only after thorough examination.

The caution and restraint exercised by those who recommend the utilization of traditional medicine together with modern scientific medicine indicates their determination not to abandon the scientific approach. Mshiu listed among the requirements for cooperation between traditional and modern medicine certain changes to which the traditional healer must agree.[59] His past activities in seclusion and isolation and the use of secrecy in his manipulations have aroused the suspicion of the trained doctor and the scientifically-oriented public. The potential for charlatanry in the absence of generally valid objective rules of behavior has been acknowledged. But it has also been admitted that serious healers have operated under self-imposed restrictions. The inadequacy of medical diagnosis is another serious obstacle which may be overcome if the two systems are coordinated. The question arises, however, whether a valuable factor in traditional medicine will be eliminated if the *mganga* is not permitted to use a spiritual approach to healing, apart from herbal treatment.

The *mganga* was found most useful in cases related to traditional, cultural, religious, and psychological health problems, such as excessive worries over life and death matters, and he has been credited with helping clients in psychosomatic cases.[60] Moreover, patients have testified that they have confidence in their traditional doctor and feel more at ease with him than in a modern hospital, where a regular doctor takes their personal history in the restrained and impersonal manner of the scientist. This is, of course, no argument against modern medicine, but it shows the role which the traditional healer is playing in today's society under the present conditions.

Another important argument in favor of coordinating the work of the two types of medical practitioners has been the continuing need for the expansion of rural services. If properly supervised, it is here that the traditional healer can fill a gap, supplementing the work of the medical assistant, who cannot cope with the large numbers of people in the dispensaries. This is not only true for rural districts. As Lloyd Swantz has shown, the *mganga* are playing an important role in urban centers, where it might be least expected.[61] He found in Dar es Salaam a greater need for the *mganga* than in rural districts. In the early 1970s, 700 medicine men treated 5,000 cases of sorcery a day among the Zaramo! Swantz found that the urban Zaramo, living in crowded quarters and intent on adjusting to new working habits in a new social environment, was unable to solve his frustrations and attributed his tensions to sorcery. He accused his neighbors, and the *mganga* was called to help him against people with whom he was not familiar. They did not belong to his old community and were not related by kinship. This represented a change from his former role as rural *mganga* because he now dealt with individuals or small family groups, not with a larger village community.[62] In spite of his adjustment to new urban economic and social conditions, the *mganga,* says Swantz, has remained the preserver of tradition. Such observations present a problem to those who expected that exposure to modern industrial society would automatically eliminate traditions of a preindustrial era. Modern planners in Tanzania seem to be confident that coordination of traditional medicine with the steadily (though slowly) expanding system of modern western scientific medicine does not present a danger to the latter.

To investigate the role of tradition in Tanzania, a traditional medical research unit was established in 1974 to study the role of traditional practitioners and their customs and practices. Curiously enough, this happened at the time of the formulation of the Third Five-Year Development Plan, destined to bring Tanzania closer to its goal of modernization. The research unit's program was not intended as a threat to scientific development. It hoped to clarify past misconceptions and to pave the way for the promotion of cooperation and understanding. It was admitted that there were risks in cooperation. Unscientific methods of diagnosis, the absence of statistics for the evaluation of disease, and unfamiliarity with modern scientific and technological advances, were all serious obstacles. The advocates of closer association within the medical system anticipated benefits from cooperation if modern doctors would be more tolerant.[63] They could, for instance, train the traditional healer to understand the danger of infection, the value of hygiene, and the importance of measuring the ingredients of drugs, without having to abandon traditional healing. It appears that the traditional healer has been willing to cooperate because he has nothing to lose. His clients are unlikely to abandon him. The supporters of traditional medicine emphasized the need for more trained auxiliaries and advocate the inclusion of the traditional healer in this category.[64]

But cooperation is not merely a question of manpower and practicality. Political considerations led TANU in 1974 to advocate research into traditional medicine. Healers represent a factor in society which, it was felt, had value and should not be sacrificed to modernization. Though the traditional healer is often illiterate, it has been found that educated as well as uneducated persons have sought their services as a recent field study in two villages in the Bagamoyo district has shown. The same study found, however, that modern medicine played a big role in the area, although "the concept of choice of place of treatment for certain diseases still persists."[65] Moreover, criticism in western societies of the impersonal character of the use of medical supertechnology has made developing societies aware of the danger of sudden and radical changes, however much these changes are needed.

Like other developing countries with limited industrialization and the need for technological imports, Tanzania aims at the transformation of its rural sector with the help of smaller-scale manufacturing and industrial establishments. This would still leave a large rural population, even after the expansion of education and better communications. The character of rural living in villages or ujamaas will not change suddenly, and traditional medicine may act as a cushion in absorbing the impact of the progress of modern scientific medicine.

9

CONCLUSION

For half a century, from 1920 to 1970, the goals set for the promotion of health and the prevention of disease in Kenya and Tanzania changed perceptibly. In spite of invariables dictated by objective factors that caused disease and determined prevention, the history of health and disease in the two East African countries is different in many respects from that of other African countries and the developing world as a whole.

Limited government budgets, restrictions of outside financing, slow improvement of productivity, steadily rising growth rates of the population, and internal political problems are among the causes which made the slogan of "health for everyone" more doubtful as the African nations progressed from the first decade of experimenting with independence to the second decade of continuing hopes and disillusionments. What makes the history of health and disease in eastern Africa different, however, is the particular character of its colonial inheritance, the differences in political systems established after independence, differences of climate and available raw materials, and different approaches to education (though both countries gave education priority among the many objectives they set for themselves). These and other factors influenced the strategy selected for disease control.

The key to health development, however, must be seen in the ability or inability to expand rural medicine without rejecting modern scientific medicine as practiced primarily in hospitals in urban and semi-urban centers. Both were so closely related that even when rural development was officially given priority, hospitals could not be denied appropriations, personnel, and foreign support. This had led some analysts to question the sincerity of commitments made after independence in the early sixties. A growing influence was exercised by new elistist groups of administrators, who influenced the performance of medical planners on the local level.[1]

Because the history of health and disease has evidenced the many factors to which it must be related in order to be understood, its complex character cannot be denied. Medical policies depend, for instance, on the economy of a country, the literacy rate of its population, the priority given to the goal of transforming old social structures to new socialist societies, and the flexibility of planners in making concessions to tradition. All these factors show the historical relevance of the medical theme in modern African history.

Both Kenya and Tanzania accepted the social impact of health promotion and disease control as a major factor in any development program; this did not mean, however, that they arrived at the same conclusions in designing their health policies. The emphasis on social issues in medicine appears more evident in Tanzania because of the *ujamaa* program. Tanzania's commitment to a socialist society, however, has not led automatically to a consistent application of socialism when administrative, ideological, and traditional obstacles arose.

In a recent well-documented study, Dean McHenry has analyzed the implementation of the principle of socialist rural living in ujamaas after the Arusha Declaration of 1967.[2] When, after an initial experimental period, peasants were asked to move to new ujamaas and assume cooperative community production, expected levels of peasant movement and of production were not reached. Under the new Villages and Ujamaa Act of 1975, a broader village scheme was introduced that permitted both communal ujamaa production and individual peasant agriculture. By 1977, 91.3 percent of the peasants had moved to the new type of ujamaa villages.[3] McHenry pointed out that although the original ujamaa plan for community-directed agricultural production was amended in 1975 to be acceptable to the majority of peasants, villagization has led to improvements in the peasants' way of life. As a byproduct of villagization, the peasants received a better water supply and better health and education facilities. This leads us to the point stressed above.[4] In spite of different ideological goals and disagreement (even within the party) on how to apply socialist standards in a poor country, the major post-independence objective of bringing more and better health facilities to the rural population was continued even though the timetable had to be adjusted and manpower training and personnel increases had to be reduced when cost and production-related items in the development program affected health funds. In 1976, for instance, the minister of health reported that only 15 new health centers and 89 dispensaries had been completed, instead of 25 health centers per year and 100 dispensaries as the Plan had targeted through the period to 1980. The unavailability of building material, transport difficulties, and poor construction capacity were to be blamed, according to Minister of Health Leader Sterling.

Ten years after the Arusha Declaration, the achievements of the health sector were examined by officials, and it was found in general that progress in the right direction had been made. "After seventeen years of Uhuru [independence], one can confidently say Tanzania's policies towards building a healthy nation are promising," wrote Isaac Mruma in the *Daily News* of Dar es Salaam in December 1977.[5] The article singled out the achievements in rural medicine, the continuation of scientific research, including the old Amani Center left over from the East African Community, the containment of tropical disease, and the increasing use made of rural medical facilities by the population at large. There were 767 doctors in Tanzania in 1977, of whom 440 were Tanzanians. Similarly, the medical auxiliary personnel had increased to 1,393 rural medical aides, though still short of the goal of 2,800 set for 1980. The goal of 50,000 people per health center appeared unattainable by 1980. Among the "anomalies" mentioned by Mruma were two items not limited to Tanzania alone but characteristic of many third world countries:

the nearly 120,000 persons under age five dying annually from malnutrition and post-natal complications and infections, and he listed perhaps still a greater anomaly, the 150 children dying every day from malnutrition. These problems cannot be solved by the health services of one country in isolation or even in conjunction with the department of agriculture responsible for food production. These are political, managerial and social problems just as much as they are problems of medicine.

As far as the quality of medical services is concerned, there are some critics even among the medical community in Tanzania; these critics know, however, that the qualitative and quantitative output of the services cannot be pushed ahead in isolation. Much depends on the simultaneous implementation of the major objectives in the Development Plans of the 1970s. These objectives include better distribution of facilities and supplies and the expansion of roads to the less populated areas, factors mentioned by McHenry in connection with rural development, and by the ministers of health in their annual budget messages.[6] The philosophy and social interpretation of health and disease has penetrated all areas of Tanzania's economy, its social, political and scientific advance, and its attitude toward modern technology as well as traditionalism.

Major goals in Kenya's health policy were not too different from those of Tanzania, but their implementation showed a different character. The right of health for every citizen and acceptance of rural medicine as a priority are two basic principles which were formulated in the sixties and then incorporated into development planning. Hospital-oriented medical care is still playing an important role in Kenya today; a changeover to a network of rural health centers was officially accepted in 1971 and vigorously implemented in the seventies. The basic questions regarding society's responsibility for health improvement and its role in village resettlement for health purposes were answered in a different way. There was more caution in debating the wisdom or feasibility of expanding the health system before the basis for development had been secured. Once the decision was made to set up a network of rural health centers and dispensaries with larger responsibilities than they had had prior to independence or in the early sixties, a substantial program for training doctors and auxiliaries was set up and coordinated with other departments of government in 1970. The close relationship between health and socio-economic planning was recognized, and machinery for interagency collaboration was set up.[7] The success of the program has not solely depended on funds from internal sources and foreign donors but more decisively, perhaps, on its vigorous enforcement through coordination with other branches of government. There is an awareness of the danger of overbureaucratization. There is a pragmatic sobriety in the shaping and formulating of the health structure that characterizes Kenya's health administration.[8] It is Kenya's version of primary health care.[9]

From a long-range perspective, the history of health and disease in eastern Africa between 1920 and 1970 shows continuity as well as contrasting phases. The return of the African Carrier Corps in 1918 taught the British administrators a shocking lesson. There was a group of men that had given the British army vital support and had proven its ability to serve not only as carriers but also as a medical-technical auxiliary. The notion was accepted in the 1920s that Africans in the rural areas needed more medical care, better education, and an opportunity to improve their lives. It took another ten years to formulate plans for the development of these men and those who came after them. Finally, the formation of viable schemes to organize an African rural medical auxiliary service began to take shape during the last decade before independence.[10]

The essential difference between colonial medical planning at its most enlightened stage in the 1950s and the national planning of Kenya and Tanzania after 1961 lies in the following: while colonial government recognized the necessity of rural medicine in eastern Africa after 1920 and especially in the 1950s, it was natural that priority be given to London's immediate concerns. British development plans for East Africa before independence were similar to those presented after 1961, especially in Tanzania. The combination, however, of a new national awareness, ambitious professional goals, and the determination to create a better and healthier society in their own country, changed the character of the public health movement in the post-independence years. It provided an urgency and a direction which it did not have before. It also opened up new problems. No longer was western expertise the exclusive aim to strive for. There was no lessening of the desire to make use of technological progress and scientific advance,[11] but there is a growing awareness that customs, cultural differences, and human behavior are basic ingredients in medical progress; this explains the interest in traditional medicine, quite apart from the economic argument that the traditional healer can supplement the auxiliary medical services.

In spite of their orientation toward the practical needs of basic health services during the first fifteen years after independence, Kenya and Tanzania did not neglect medical research. Research programs started on a modest scale under the East African Medical Research Council of the East African Community. By the time of its dissolution in 1977, the Council had established a network of research projects throughout the region.[12] For a period of over ten years, Kenya and Tanzania were able to maintain theoretical and applied research in tropical disease, tuberculosis and natural resources. Only three years after the end of the East African Community, the tradition of medical scientific research was resumed with the convening of the First Annual Medical Scientific Conference in Nairobi in January 1980. Though no longer funded by the combined resources of the three East African countries, medical scientific research was proclaimed as an essential factor for the performance of medical services and the control of disease. Scientific research as well as research directed toward practical goals in society was given a new start. Its reappearance in spite of political tensions in eastern Africa enhances confidence in the continuing policies of socio-economic development of the area.

The commitment by government to support research was demonstrated by the enactment of the Science and Technology Act of 1979, followed by the establishment of a National Council of Science and Technology, and by research institutes in the appropriate ministries.[13] The Kenya government committed itself to an allocation of 1 percent of its GNP for research and pledged KSh 6 million for medical research during the 1979-83 Development Plan.

Medical research in developing countries, however, must carefully define its special tasks, as Dr. A. M. Nhonoli of the University of Dar es Salaam emphasized at the same meeting.[14] He stressed that such research must examine why many projects in rural areas have failed in the past and whether their failure was due to the inappropriateness of a technology not compatible with the particular conditions in a certain environment. Scientific research in eastern Africa, therefore, must be selective, even if a choice has to be made at the expense of basic research. Nhonoli recommended adding a fourth category to the three accepted categories of research in eastern Africa; in addition to biomedical laboratory-based research, clinical hospital-based research, and medico-social community research, research on appropriate technology should be added.[15] The need for this kind of research has also been noted by other medical planners in Africa and in the western world, and it is particularly justifiable under economic conditions which prevent many developing countries from upgrading the technology of their medical institutions.

At a time when modern medical institutions in the western world have become more conscious of the human factor in the doctor-patient relationship, Africans may be able to avoid some of the excesses of technical advances without losing sight of scientific goals; but their principal concern for the foreseeable future will remain the sustained drive to help improve the medico-social condition of the rural population. Several statements by health officials in 1976 and 1978 support this conclusion. Tanzania's minister of health said in his budget speech to the House in 1976: "The future of the health services of Tanzania will, to a large extent, depend on medical skill of medical assistants and rural medical aides. These cadres are the mainstay of the front-line health services, especially in the rural health services." He also referred to the "bare facts" of the great human problem, a population of 15 million people, threatened by "malnutrition, by lack of clean water, by lack of good housing and adequate sanitation, and by all the fruits of poverty." In addition to these formidable obstacles, the shortage of medical manpower continued. In spite of the expanded training programs during the period 1967-1977, there was still only one doctor for 23,000 people in 1977 and one dispensary for five villages.[16]

Kenya's deputy director of health made similar points in an address to the International Conference on Primary Health at Alma Ata, U.S.S.R., in 1978.[17] He presented the concepts and structure of Kenya's health services in 1978 and referred to the still-remaining health problems. Kenya aimed at health units with a maximum of 50,000 people. In these units, specially selected and trained health workers would be able to identify and define the problems of the various regions. Teams under public health workers, agricultural technicians, and educators trained in family health would be enlisted to help in the control of disease, poverty, and ignorance through the regions. Although the identification of goals is only one of the many steps toward health improvement and better living conditions, without the commitment to these goals, development planning would become meaningless. Making the right choices does not necessarily imply that the desired results will be obtained. Without the right choices, however, the selection of goals remains an idle dream.

APPENDIX

The objectives of the Tanzanian development plans between 1950 and 1980 reflect the changing concepts of government, the transition to new social systems and the resulting adjustments to different economic priorities. Some of the major principles of ecomonic planning and selected statistics on medicine and rural living are presented here to substantiate the more general presentation of the book.

SELECTED PRINCIPLES OF THE DEVELOPMENT PLANS

Ten Year Development and Welfare Plan for Tanganyika, 1947-1956

This plan, revised after only three years, accepted the premise that economic or productive development should take prior place to social services. It opted for the growth of the sisal industry, the expansion of mining and the promotion of commercial and industrial activity (Plan, p. 4). It decided to use the colonial development and welfare funds primarily for the strengthening of the infrastructure of the Territory. It did not effect a change in the social structure of the African urban and rural districts.

Breakdown of allocation under the Revised Plan of 1950 (Plan, p. 10):

	£	%
Conservation and Development of Natural Resources	4,355,191	17.8
Communications	8,783,000	35.9
Social Services	2,934,000	12.0
Township Development	3,573,000	14.6
Public Buildings	3,480,000	14.2
African Urban Housing	1,230,000	5.0
Miscellaneous	115,000	0.5

Development Plan for Tanganyika, 1961/62-1963/64
Dar es Salaam, 1961

Based on a World Bank Mission report submitted in 1960, the Three Year Plan became operative five months before independence. It called for a more rapid growth of the economy, and proposed to finance the development of agriculture, the improvement of communications and the development of secondary and technical education financed by capital from external and internal borrowing. As Pratt pointed out, the Three Year Development Plan was not an essay toward the realization of a socialistic state. (Pratt: *The Critical Phase in Tanzania, 1945-1968*, p. 96). The main theme of the Plan was the laying of the foundation for future growth. The statistics bear out these assumptions (The Three Year Development Plan, Smith, Readings, p. 357):

Ministry	£ 000	%
Prime Minister	1,252	5.2
Agriculture	5,737	24.0
Communications, Power and Works	6,900	28.0
Education	3,270	13.7
Commerce and Industry	1,095	4.6
Local Government	1,244	5.2
Home Affairs	2,100	9.1
Health and Labor	954	4.0
Lands and Surveys	1,298	5.4
	23,000	100.0

Tanganyika Five Year Plan for Economic and Social Development, 1964-1969

Among the principles stated in the Five Year Development Plan were:

1. The commitment to the philosophy of African Socialism based on a more equitable distribution of wealth.
2. Raising the per capita income from £19.6 in 1962 to £85 in 1980.
3. Educational and political measures to change the attitude of the rural population toward economic growth.

Several of the targets of this Plan were not reached. This was due in part to inaccuracies in the available statistical information. The population was not growing at a rate of 2.2 percent as assumed, but at a rate of 2.7 percent. More important, however, was the impact of political changes such as the mutiny of Tanzanian soldiers in 1964, the merger of Tanganyika and Zanzibar into the United Republic of Tanzania in 1964, and the Arusha Declaration of 1967. Energies and efforts needed for the success of the development plan were absorbed by political and administrative changes.

Second Five-Year Plan for Economic and Social Development in Tanzania, 1969-1974

Several changes in the objectives and in strategy were made in this Plan. It incorporated the following five principles:

1. Social equality, i.e., the attempt to spread the benefits of development widely throughout society.
2. *Ujamaa,* i.e., the emphasis on economic development in rural areas through cooperatives and collectives.
3. Self-reliance through the maximum mobilization of domestic resources.
4. Economics and social transformation with the aid of an accelerated expansion of Tanzania's productive capacity.
5. African economic integration in the hope of extending economic cooperation with other African states.

Impact of Development Plans on Medicine:
Tanzania During the Colonial Period, and after 1961

Government Budgets for Health Expenditure in Tanzania

1950-1956 £1,780,000	Proposed Budget, (Revised Development and Welfare Plan, DSM, Government Printer, 1951)
1961-1964 £954,000	Development Plan for Tanganyika, 1961/62-1962/63 (DSM, Government Printer, 1962)
1964-1969 £13,988,000	An Outline of Medical Development, 1964-1969 (Dar es Salaam, Ministry of Health, 1964)

Development of Rural Health Centers:
The Colonial Period in Tanzania

1926	The beginning of a rural dispensary system. Tribal dressers with three months of training.
1930	Training period for dressers extended to eighteen months to three years in four schools at Tabora, Misoma, Bukoba, and Tukuyu.
1945	Training concentrated in one school at Mwanza.
1949	The rural medical stations are placed under medical inspection controlled by district medical officers.
1951	Rural medical aids grouped according to training: Grade I – Educational standard X, three years of training as medical aide Grade II – Educational standard VIII, not less than two years of training as medical aide Grade III– Less than the minimum education for Grades I and II, little or no medical training

Rural Dispensaries in 1950

Number of Stations	Rural Medical Aides	Total Patient Attendance
416	445	3,655,248

("Rural Health Services." TNA File 13350. Dar es Salaam)

Rural Medical Facilities, Tanzania, 1961-1980

	1961	*1969*	*1974*	*1980*
Dispensaries	736	1,362	1,500	2,500 planned
Rural Health Centers	22	50	100	300 planned
	1961	*1969*	*1972*	*1974-80*
Medical Assistants	200	250	335	210-250 planned intake per year
	1961	*1969*	*1973-4*	*1974-80*
Rural Medical Aides	200	450	578	560 planned intake per year

Functions of Rural Health Centers:

To serve a population of approximately 50,000 persons.

To provide supervision of dispensaries in its area, to organize preventive campaigns, environmental sanitation, and nutrition among others.

Functions of Dispensaries:

To provide service for communities of approximately 10,000 people.

The minimum standards, not considered satisfactory in 1964, subject to continued revision and improvement.

(Tanzania Second Five-Year Development Plan, Dar es Salaam, XI; Health Budget Speech by Minister for Health, A. H. Mwiny, 1973-7, Dar es Salaam; Gish, Oscar, *Planning the Health Sector,* London: 1975, p. 79.)

Development Planning in Kenya

Sessional Paper No. 10

Kenya's First Development Plan after independence, published as *Sessional Paper No. 10* in 1965, accepted the principle that African Socialism as defined by Kenya's party, KANU, would be the basis for the implementation of development. This gave the government a broad umbrella under which to formulate the immediate goals for the first stage of development. Among them were the growth of the public and cooperative sector of the economy, the role of self-help or *Harambee,* provisions for a broad system of education, the Africanization of the economy and the development of the welfare services. Human health, it was said in the Plan, had a major role to play in economic development. "There [was] a direct relationship between the health of the population and its productivity." (Plan, p. 107)

Development Planning and Public Health

The Throughton Report of 1946 proposed that all services, personal and non-personal, preventive and curative, be placed under the direction of the central government. After 1963, these broad principles continued to guide health development in Kenya. A more specific assignment of tasks, however, and the definition of goals in a changing political and economic climate, led to the reorganization of health policy after 1970.

The Health Development Plan for 1970-1974 identified the main problems as the shortage of trained staff, and the inadequate and poor facilities. The need for the expansion of health centers was seen. They were described as the backbone of the health services, providing basic services in rural areas where 90 percent of the people lived.

The 1974-1978 Kenya Development Plan gave special consideration to the rural health services program with an upgrading schedule for the expansion of rural health services by 1978.

Rural Development in Kenya

Projections of Expenditure in Health, 1963-1984 (K£million)

FY	Government as Whole		Ministry of Health		Percent of Total	
	Recurrent	Development	Recurrent	Development	Recurrent	Development
1962-63	28.2	11.1	1.9	0.36	6.3	3.2
1967-68	47.9	20.1	3.7	0.84	7.8	4.2
1971-72	92.5	51.5	6.3	2.8	6.8	5.5
1972-73 projected	92.9	66.0	7.5	3.62	7.6	5.5
1979-80 projected	199.0	229.7	19.3	18.3	--	--

(Ministry of Health, Proposal for the Improvement of Rural Health Services, Nairobi, 1972).

Rural Medical Facilities (Types as Listed in 1974-78 Development Plan, p. 454)

Health Center

One preventive clinic block with supporting services. An in-patient block with twelve beds. Staff: one medical assistant, four community nurses, one health assistant, two family-planning field workers, one statistical clerk and attendant staff.

Health Sub-Center

Similar clinics and supporting services, no in-patient block. One medical assistant, two community nurses, one health assistant, one or two family-planning field workers and attending staff.

Dispensary

One clinic block and service facilities. Staffed by health assistant, community nurse and staff.

Manpower requirements in health facilities (rural)

FY	Medical Assistants	Community Nurses	Health Assistants
1972-73	24	100	40
1975-76	33	147	66
1979-80	48	215 projection	77

Population per health center

	Centers	Rural Population	Rural Population Per Center
1972	162	9,862,797	60,881
1984	244	--	66,000 projection

Goal: One health center per 20,000 population.

Kenya: Population Growth Rates

Year	Population	Growth Rate (%) Between Years Shown
1931	3,981,000	2.0
1941	4,853,000	2.0
1948	5,405,966	––
1951	6,211,000	2.5
1961	8,346,000	3.0
1962	8,636,263	3.2
1969	10,942,705	3.3
1971	11,524,000	3.4
1974	12,934,000	3.5

(Kenya Development Plan, 1974-78, Ministry of Health, Nairobi, 1974.)

NOTES

INTRODUCTORY REMARKS

1. I am aware that E. A. Brett in his book *Colonialism and Underdevelopment in East Africa* criticizes the Development Act of 1929 as misdirected, since it was conceived as a measure to reduce unemployment in Britain and stimulate the home economy. See Chapter 1 below.

2. Since the dissolution of the East African Community in 1977, Kenya and Tanzania prefer to be treated as separate entities. Though different in character, especially as a result of internal changes since independence, there are overriding characteristics which lend themselves to comparative treatment.

CHAPTER 1: DEVELOPMENT IN COLONIAL EAST AFRICA AFTER 1920: THE FORMULATION OF GOALS

1. Statements on development and policies promoting development may be found in Annual Medical Reports of Kenya, Uganda and Tanganyika Territory, 1920-1940; A number of Command Papers, 1923-1940, such as "Indians in Kenya," Memorandum on Native Policy in East Africa, Cmd. 1922, 1923; "Future Policy in regard to Eastern Africa," Cmd. 2904, 1927; "Report of the Commission on Closer Union of the Dependencies in Eastern Africa, 1928-1929," Cmd. 3234, 1929; "Memorandum on Native Policy in East Africa," Cmd. 3573, 1930; "Certain Questions in Kenya," Report by Lord Moyne, 1932, Cmd. 4093, 1932. Also L. S. Amery, *My Political Life,* vol. 2, ch. XI. And the specific reports on development acts, 1930, 1940, 1945 as well as the reports by the Advisory Committee on Colonial Development, 1930-1940.

2. See E. A. Brett, *Colonialism and Underdevelopment in East Africa,* p. 129.

3. See Report of the East African Commission, 1925, Cmd. 2387 p. 38 on the "contact theory" and p. 186 the "tribal control theory." See also John W. Cell, *By Kenya Possessed, The Correspondence of Norman Leys and J. H. Oldham, 1918-1926,* appendix J. H. Oldham, "A Note on the Report of the East African Commission," 1926, pp. 295,316.

4. Memorandum on Native Policy in East Africa, Cmd. 3573, 1930, pp. 5, 7.

5. Brett, op. cit., ch. 4, British Unemployment and Colonial Aid, pp. 115-140.

6. Ibid, pp. 131, ff.

7. Cmd. 3540, 1929-30. First Interim Report of the Colonial Development Advisory Committee, appendix, p. 20. Under the Act funds were available as capital grants, free interest grants, and loans. The Colonial Development Advisory Committee consisted "entirely of men with interest in business and experience of organizations connected with colonial development." Brett, op. cit., p. 134. See also appendix for statistics on total allocations.

8. Cmd. 3268, 1928-29, appendix p. 20 and 73.

9. See Brett's extensive documentation of the Colonial Development Act of 1929 with references to Cabinet Papers, speeches and the official development literature. Brett, op. cit., part II, ch. 5.

10. Quoted in Brett, p. 129. In this context it is worth remembering that from the seventeenth century onwards, the colonial empires of Spain and Portugal had made serious mistakes in their trading policies. They learned the hard way that their undue concentration on profit in the interest of the homeland stunted the growth of their American possessions and forced them to import slave labor which ultimately proved to be against their own interest. Similar experiences were made by the British and French in the eighteenth century. At the beginning of the twentieth century, however, though official policy did not change noticeably, statements were made on the need to develop the indigenous populations and more serious suggestions in this respect were included in the formulation of policy by 1920.

11. See, for instance, the Hilton Young Report on Closer Union of 1928-1929 and Colonial Development Committee report of 1930, which argue extensively on areas of development applicable to African life. The members of the Colonial Development Advisory Committee found it difficult to select development schemes which would fit the direction in which development was expected to go.

12. Hilton Young Report, p. 15.

13. "Certain Questions in Kenya." Report by Financial Commissioner Lord Moyne, Cmd. 4093, 1932, p. 9.

14. First Interim Report of the Colonial Development Advisory Committee, Cmd. 3540, 1930, p. 17.

15. Colonial Development Advisory Committee, Cmd. 6298, 1941, p. 11.

16. Brett, op. cit., p. 136.

17. First Interim Report of the Colonial Development Advisory Committee, Cmd. 3540, p. 18 and Brett, op. cit., pp. 135-137.

18. Colonial Development Advisory Committee, Cmd. 6298, 1941, p. 9.

19. Colonial Administration and Welfare, Cmd. 6713, 1945, p. 2.

20. Cmd. 410, 1939-1940, "Statement of Policy on Colonial Development and Welfare," p. 5

CHAPTER 2: MEDICINE AND DEVELOPMENT PLANNING: THE COLONIAL PERIOD

1. See, for instance, Paul Streeten, "Changing Perceptions of Development,"

Finance and Development, vol. 14, pp. 14-16 (1977), J. M. Lee, *Colonial Development and Good Government: A Study of Ideas Expressed by the British Official Classes in Planning Decolonization, 1939-1964,* Oxford University Press, 1967; Cyril E. Black, *The Dynamics of Modernization,* Princeton, 1966; Colin Leys, "The Political Climate for Economic Development," *African Affairs,* 1966, pp. 55-60. Denis Goulet, *The Cruel Choice: A New Concept in the Theory of Development,* 1975; Vincente Navarro, "The Underdevelopment of Health or the Health of Underdevelopment: An Analysis of the Distribution of Health Resources in Latin America," *International Journal of Health Services,* vol. 4, no. 1, 1974.

2. See Chapter 1.

3. "Future Policy in Regard to East Africa," Great Britain, Sessional Papers, Cmd. 2904, p. 2, London, 1927.

4. "Report of the Commission on Closer Union of the Dependencies in Eastern and Central Africa, 1928-1929," p. 60, Cmd. 3234.

5. "Report of Sir Samuel Wilson on his Visit to East Africa, 1929," p. 31, Cmd. 3378.

6. E. A. Brett, *Colonialism and Underdevelopment in East Africa,* p. 136.

7. "Colonial Development and Welfare," Cmd. 6113, 1945-46, p. 2.

8. This episode is described in TNA File 26854, "Proposed new School of Medicine and Hygiene," Dar es Salaam, issued by the Central Development Committee, 1939. That the project was seriously considered by Government is also indicated by an inquiry in the House of Commons on March 5, 1930. Ormsby-Gore asked Under-Secretary of State for the Colonies where the medical training school was to be established, what grades of assistants, and for what periods of time were to be trained and what service—government or mission—they would enter after training. See Great Britain, House of Commons, March 5, 1930, p. 420.

9. TNA, File 26854, pp. 79-80.

10. Ibid., p. 80.

11. Ibid., p. 82.

12. TNA, File 26854, Director of Medical Services, Dar es Salaam to Secretary, The Central Development Committee, Dar es Salaam, 22nd March, 1939.

13. Ibid., p. 2. Population density varied widely. In Lake Province it was 28 per square mile. In fertile areas it could reach as high as 1,000 per square mile.

14. Ibid., pp. 5-6.

15. Selected statistics indicate the inadequacies.

Province	MO	MMP	SAS	Population	Pop. per MO	Pop. per MO & MMP & SAS
Central	2	4	4	545,260	272,630	54,526
Eastern	6	3	12	639,616	106,603	30,458
Lake	5	4	8	1,461,192	292,238	85,952
Tanga	3	2	7	352,986	117,662	29,415

Note: MO=Medical Officer; MMP=Missionary Medical Practitioner; SAS=Sub-Assistant Surgeon.

Ibid., p. 6.

16. Ibid., p. 7.

17. TNA, File 26854, Memorandum on Tuberculosis in Tanganyika Territory, pp. 4, 6, 7.

18. Memorandum on the Future Development of the Medical Services of Tanganyika Territory by the Director of Medical Services, 1943, Dar es Salaam, 1944. One should be careful, however, in interpreting numbers of doctors stationed in sleeping sickness territory and malaria-infested areas. I am grateful to an explanation by Dr. H. G. Calwell, former sleeping sickness officer in Tanzania between 1930 and 1949. He pointed out to me that epidemics did not always occur at the same time everywhere. The doctors were peripatetic, he wrote, and worked where they were needed and could cope with the load of patients with the help of African assistants. Personal communication to author, March 1979.

19. Ibid., p. 2.

20. Legislative Council of Tanganyika, "A Review of the Medical Policy of Tanganyika," Government Printer, Dar es Salaam, 1949.

21. Memorandum on the Future Development, p. 2.

22. P. A. T. Sneath to Chief Secretary to the Government, Dar es Salaam, TNA File 12602, vol. II, 12th December 1947, with memorandum on the Village Dispensaries.

23. For a more detailed evaluation of Sneath's history of the village dispensaries, see Chapter 3 below. It was Sneath's intention to activate and revitalize a stalemated service. He did give credit to its achievements in spite of long periods of economic world crises.

24. TNA, File 12602, vol. II, 12 December 1947.

25. The detail of his rejection of an expanded dispensary service under the conditions of 1947 is discussed in Chapter 3.

26. TNA, File 12602, "History of Tribal Dresser System," 1947, p. 9.

27. Ibid., p. 10.

28. Legislative Council of Tanganyika, "A Review of the Medical Policy of Tanganyika," Government Printer, Dar es Salaam, 1949.

29. Ibid., p. 2.

30. "The Colonial Empire," Cmd. 7167, 1946-47, p. 28.

31. See Chapter 1, p. 5.

32. "The Colonial Empire," Cmd. 7167, p. 28.

CHAPTER 3: RURAL MEDICAL SERVICES: THE COLONIAL PERIOD

1. TNA, File 13350, "A Rural Dispensary System," vol. III. Historical, p. 1.

2. See Ann Beck, *Medicine and Society in Tanzania,* p. 41, ff.

3. See, for instance, the correspondence between medical directors Scott and Sneath and Provincial Commissioners and the Secretariat in Dar es Salaam.

4. Principal Medical Officer John Gilks, Annual Medical Report, Colony and Protectorate of Kenya, 1921 (1922), p. 17.

5. In *Rural Health Development in Tanzaania,* Van Gorcum, 1976, Dr. G. M.

van Etten traced the history of rural health policy in Tanzania from the 1926 directive on rural dispensaries to the system as it existed before independence and made two major factors responsible for its failure: (1) political and medical factors, such as the post-war trend toward a more humane colonial administration and the recurring medical emergencies, and (2) economic factors such as the limited amount in taxes available to the Native Authorities. I shall take issue with these arguments below. See also Dr. G. Jansen, *The Doctor-Patient Relationship in an African Tribal Society,* Van Gorcum 1973.

6. TNA, File 11675, Annual Report Central Province, January 1928, pp. 20-22 See also ibid., 1929, p. 282. Not only acceptance of dispensaries by Africans, but also the performance of dressers was praised.

7. Ibid., 29 February, 1933, p. 50.

8. TNA, File 12602, vol. II, Village Dispensaries, maintained by Native Treasuries. 1947, pp. 2, 3.

	1926	1927	1928	1930
Tribal dressers	0	90	147	288
Total attendance	0	2,000	?	352,423

9. TNA, File 12602, B. "History of the Tribal Dresser System," 1947, p. 4.

10. See Chapter 2 above.

11. TNA, File 12602, History, p. 9.

12. Chapter 2 above.

13. TNA, File 12602, History, p. 9.

14. See G. M. van Etten, *Rural Health Development in Tanzania,* ch. 2. He correctly relates the NA ability to raise sufficient taxes, within the limitations granted by the colonial administration to the strengthening of NA administered rural dispensaries. These were, however, only some of the reasons for stunting the growth of the dispensaries before 1939.

15. TNA, File 12602, History, p. 12.

16. TNA, File 13350, "Rural Health Service," pp. 1, 2.

17. Ibid., pp. 3-7. The previously established grading system for rural aides was to be kept. Grades I and II remained the same, whereas Grade III was downgraded. Its staff would have an education below standard VIII and only some form of medical training.

18. See Appendix.

19. *Revised Development and Welfare Plan for Tanganyika, 1950-1956.* Government Printer, Dar es Salaam, 1951, p. 9.

20. "Plan," pp. 3, 34.

21. Annual Medical Report, Kenya, John L. Gilks, 1926, p. 48.

22. Lord Hailey, *An African Survey,* 1956, pp. 446-447.

23. *Health and Disease in Kenya,* L. C. Vogel ed., East African Literature Bureau, Nairobi, 1974; see article by Ann Beck, "History of Medicine and Health Services in Kenya, 1900 to 1950," pp. 91-105.

24. A. R. Patterson, Annual Medical Reports, 1933-1937, Medical Department, Kenya Colony.

25. Colony and Protectorate of Kenya, Medical, Annual Report, 1953, pp. 14-15.

26. Ibid., 1955, p. 11.

27. Ministry of Health and Housing, Annual Report for 1962, p. 1.

28. See above, p. 19.

CHAPTER 4: RESEARCH AND DEVELOPMENT: THE COLONIAL PERIOD

1. For a more detailed presentation of the start of scientific research in eastern Africa, see Ann Beck, "Medical and Scientific Research in East Africa. Progress and Impediments, 1900-1961." ATTI Del XXI Congresso Internazionale Di Storia Della Medicina, Siena, 1958, pp. 1063-1073 and idem, "Scientific Medical Research and the Control of Parasitic Disease in East Africa," East African Medical Research Council, 23rd Annual Scientific Conference, East African Literature Bureau, Nairobi, Kenya, 1978.

2. ATTI, p. 1065.

3. Ibid.

4. For further detail on the establishment of the East African Research Bureau and the East African Research Council, see Ann Beck, *A History of the British Medical Administration of East Africa,* 1900-1950, Harvard University Press, pp. 185-197.

5. After 1961, the Bureau became the East African Medical Research Council which ceased operations with the dissolution of the East African Community in 1977.

6. TNA, File 34051, Organization of Scientific Research and Research Services in the Colonial Empire, 1947-1951, E. B. Worthington, pp. 181-182.

7. On the history of medical administration, see Ann Beck, *A History of the British Medical Administration in East Africa* and idem, *Society and Medicine in Tanganyika,* Transactions of the American Philosophical Society, Philadelphia, 1977. Also, T. W. J. Schulpen, *Integration of Church and Government Medical Services in Tanzania,* Nairobi, Kenya, 1975.

8. To describe the policy of procrastination in research development in East Africa as the logical result of "colonialism" would not be helpful in a study which attempts to unravel the concurrence and interaction of circumstantial causes, economic choices, actual human needs, medical necessities and social traditions.

9. R. I. M. Swynnerton, "A Plan to Intensify the Development of African Agriculture in Kenya," 1955, Nairobi, Government Printer.

10. Annual Medical Report for 1926, Government Printer, Nairobi, p. 10.

11. Annual Medical Report for 1936, ibid., pp. 4, 5.

12. Annual Report of the East African Council for Medical Research, 1954-1955, East African High Commission, Nairobi, 1955, pp. 11-12, 27.

13. Michael C. Latham, "Priorities for Nutrition and Health Programs in Africa," African Studies Association 19th Annual Meeting, Boston, Mass., 1976, p. 2.

14. Alan L. Sorokin, *Health Economics in Developing Countries,* D. C. Heath, 1976.

CHAPTER 5: TRANSITION TO INDEPENDENCE AND THE CONTINUITY OF MEDICAL GOALS

1. *Revised Development and Welfare Plan for Tanganyika,* Government Printer, Dar es Salaam, 1951, p. 1.

2. The Plan distinguished between the original Ten Year model set up in 1947 and the revised model of 1950. What had originally seemed to be desirable for approaching the full potential of the Territory was no longer correct. More emphasis was placed on conservation and development of natural resources, communications, public buildings, agriculture and urban as well as African urban housing.

Selected items from the revised totals

	£	%
Conservation and development of natural resources	4,365,191	17.8
Social Services	2,934,000	12.0
Buildings and Works	3,480,000	14.2
African Urban Housing	1,230,000	5.0

The Social Services were broken down into three items: medical (mostly hospital building), education (teacher training, secondary education and primary education) and rural development as part of social development.

3. Lord Hailey, *An African Survey,* 1956, p. 1325.

4. See above, ch. 3.

5. Quoted in Cranford Pratt, *The Critical Phase in Tanzania,* 1945-1968, p. 16. See also critique of development acts in ch. 2 above.

6. Sir Andrew Cohen, *British Policy in Changing Africa,* p. 88.

7. Pratt, *The Critical Phase,* pp. 47, ff. I am aware that this emphasis on the role of middle-level officials may be misinterpreted as not giving sufficient credit to the African strategy of President Nyerere and TANU. I agree, however, with Pratt's distinction between the thinking of the top echelon in Dar es Salaam and the officers in the field who saw African affairs from a different angle.

8. Revised Development and Welfare Plan for Tanganyika, p. 2.

9. See Chapter 2 above, pp. 10-11.

10. A Plan for the Development of Medical Services in Tanganyika, 1956-1961 (hereafter "Plan"), Government Printer, Dar es Salaam, 1956, p. 4.

11. Ibid., pp. 109-110.

12. Ibid., pp. 6-8.

13. Ibid.

14. Richard M. Titmuss, *The Health Services of Tanganyika* (Titmuss Report), 1963, pp. 31, 32.

15. The Mau Mau movement, organized in 1947 as a secret society bound by oath to drive the Europeans out of their land, became a violent force in the early 1950s. The Mau Mau Emergency was declared by the Government in 1953.

16. Government of Kenya, Ministry of Health and Housing, Annual Report, 1962, p. 1.

17. Ibid., pp. 1, 2 and Ann Beck, "History of Medicine and Health Services in Kenya," *Health and Disease in Kenya,* East African Literature Bureau, 1974, pp. 91-106.

18. The Medical Report for 1953 stated that even in the United Kingdom local authorities found it hard to keep their sanitary inspectors up to strength. Annual Report, Medical Department, Colony and Protectorate of Kenya, 1953, p. 19.

19. There is an ambiguity in the use of the term rural health centers. District and Provincial hospitals were classed as main health centers from which radiated a supervisory staff to control the "ever-growing network" of rural health centers. A more precise classification of health centers and their role was given in 1972 in *Proposals for the Improvement of Rural Health Services and the Development of Rural Health Training Centers in Kenya,* Ministry of Health, 1972.

20. In 1962, there were 140 health centers and 20 sub-centers as against nil in 1946. Government had increased its capacity from 3,000 hospital beds in 1946 to 6,424 in 1962. These increases were achieved in spite of a population growth from 5.4 million in 1948 to 8.67 million in 1962. Kenya Medical Report, pp. 1, 2.

21. Problems in medical administration and financing stemming from constitutional changes will be discussed in Chapter 6.

CHAPTER 6: DEVELOPMENT AND HEALTH POLICY IN TANZANIA

1. Hadley E. Smith, ed., *Readings on Economic Development and Administration in Tanzania* (hereafter quoted as *Readings*), "Development Plan for Tanganyika 1961/62-1963/64," Dar es Salaam, 1962, pp. 348-356.

2. Ibid., "Tanganyika Five Year Plan for Economic and Social Development," Dar es Salaam, 1964, 371.

3. The term "peasant" is used here to describe the independent agricultural cultivator living in cooperative villages or on his own small piece of land, even though some of his produce may be sold on international markets. Not only his mode of production but also his life style are different from the agricultural laborers employed on state farms or working on behalf of international companies. The distinction made in European agricultural history between peasant and farmer is not applicable to conditions in Tanzania.

4. See, for instance, L. Cliffe and J. S. Saul, *General Problems of Rural Development Policy in Tanzania,* vol. II, E. A. Publishing House, 1973.; Gavin Williams, "Taking the Part of the Peasants: Rural Development in Nigeria and Tanzania," in Gutkind and Wallerstein, eds., *The Political Economy of Contemporary Africa,* 1976; Andrew Coulson, "Agricultural Policies in Mainland Tanzania," *Review of African Political Economy,* London, 1976.

5. Philip Ehrensaft, "Polarized Accumulation and the Theory of Economic Dependence: The Implications of South African Semi-Industrial Capitalism," Gutkind and Wallerstein, op. cit. 61. Ehrensaft's analysis of the relationship between center and periphery provides a clue to one particular sector of Tanzania's agricultural society which remained remarkably unchanged under colonial rule.

6. Lionel Cliffe, "Rural Political Economy of Africa," Gutkind and Wallerstein, op. cit. 125-127.

7. Gavin Williams, "Taking the Part of the Peasants: Rural Development in Nigeria and Tanzania,", ibid., 131-154.

8. Julius Nyerere, "Presidential Circular No. 1," 1969, in Cliffe et al., *Rural Cooperation in Tanzania,* 1975, p. 27.

9. Julius K. Nyerere, "Socialism and Rural Development," in Cliffe et al., ed. *Rural Cooperation,* pp. 9, 10.

10. Dean E. McHenry, Jr., *Tanzania's Ujamaa Villages.* The Implementation of a Rural Development Strategy, Institute of International Studies, University of California, Berkeley, 1979, p. 222.

11. Vincente Navarro, "The Underdevelopment of Health or the Health of Underdevelopment: An Analysis of the Distribution of Human Health Resources in Latin America," *International Journal of Health Services,* vol. 4, no. 1, 1974, 5-27.

12. Oscar Gish, *Planning the Health Sector,* 20-24.

13. Ministry of Health, Dar es Salaam, 1964, *An Outline of Medical Development,* 1964-1969. During a visit to Dar es Salaam, I had an opportunity to talk to several members of the Medical Development Committee in 1964 and noticed their serious concern with their task of formulating plans for medical care in Tanzania while the future of the country was still uncertain.

14. Ibid., 1.

15. Ibid., 5.

16. Ibid., 11 and Gish, 20.

17. Ibid., 6.

18. Richard M. Titmuss, chairman, *The Health Services of Tanganyika,* London, 1964. The Report was commissioned by the Ministry of Health in 1961 to examine the existing organization of medical services and recommend suggestions for future expansion. It considered the financing of the services, the population factor, the rural population and the strategy of development. Titmuss deserves credit for his advocacy of preventive services in spite of the persistent need for hospitals and clinical services. The Titmuss Report had an influence on the First Five Year Plan (Etten, *Rural Health Development in Tanzania,* 1976) but according to Gish, it was not "consciously referred to by administrators" in later years.

19. *Tanganyika Five Year Plan for Economic and Social Development, 1964-1969,* Dar es Salaam, 1964. X, XXII, XXIII.

20. United Republic of Tanzania, *The Annual Plan for 1971/72,* 1971. Dar es Salaam, p. 5. The Plan has been extensively discussed by Gish, op. cit., pp. 24-31 and by Etten, op. cit., pp. 42-45. For statistics on doctors, rural centers and goals for 1974, see Appendix.

21. United Republic of Tanzania, *Tanzania Second Five Year Plan for Economic and Social Development*, 1st July, 1969-30th June, 1974, vol. I, pp. 148-165, and *Annual Plan* for 1971/73, p. 90.

22. *Annual Plan,* pp. 4, 5.

23. *Annual Medical Report,* Chief Medical Officer, 1968/69 (1970), DSM, Ministry of Health, p. 3.

24. *The Annual Plan,* 1971/72, p. 49.

25. *Five Year Plan,* 1969/74, p. 163.

26. Budget speech by the Minister for Health, Hon. A. H. Mwinyi for the Year 1973/74, pp. 1, 2.

27. Ibid., pp. 8, 9.

28. Budget Speech, Mwinyi, 1973, p. 15.

29. World Health Organization, *Tropical Diseases Today–The Challenge and the Opportunity,* Geneva, 1975, p. 5.

30. Paraphrased from WHO, "Recommendations and Report of the Planning Group of the Special Programme for Research and Training in Tropical Diseases," 1974, Geneva, p. 7.

31. For the distinction between acceptable norms of traditional healing and disreputable healers, see below chapter VIII on Traditional African Medicine.

32. Budget Speech, Minister for Health, Mwinyi, 1972, pp. 30-35 and 1973, pp. 17-18.

33. Budget Speech, Minister for Health Stirling, 1976, p. 5.

34. Ibid., p. 17.

35. See Reports on British Public Health History and recent reports on rats in major American cities.

36. Budget Speech, Minister of Health, 1976, p. 43.

37. Dr. F. D. E. Mtango, "The Role of the Doctor in Rural Health Services: Scientific Medicine Through Medical Auxiliaries," unpublished paper, 1978.

38. *Daily News,* Dar es Salaam, September 28, 1979. The statement was made at the 29th session of the World Health Organization Regional Committee for Africa, held in Maputo, Mocambique.

CHAPTER 7: RESTRUCTURING MEDICAL SERVICES IN KENYA AFTER INDEPENDENCE

1. It is not the intention to present in this chapter a study of contrasting characteristics of the two countries, describing them as socialistic, capitalistic, elitist, western or tribal. These labels will not clarify the role played by medical policy, however significant the chacteristics are.

2. See chapter 2, pp. 12-13, and ch. 5, p. 35 above.

3. See chapter 5, p. 35.

4. Government of Kenya, Ministry of Health and Housing, *Annual Report,* 1962, p. 1. Unfortunately I was unable to locate records on debates or disagreements on the Throughton Report, contrary to the lively debates in Tanzanian records on the proposals by Dr. P. T. A. Sneath between 1945 and 1947, and by Dr. Pridie in the 1950s.

5. Ibid., p. 5.

6. Ibid., pp. 2, 3. See also general evaluation of the colonial medical services in Kenya in Ann Beck, "History of Medicine and Health Services in Kenya (1900-1950)," in *Health and Disease in Kenya,* ed. L. C. Vogel and others, East African Literature Bureau 1974.

7. Reference is made here to the Ministry of Health, although its name was Ministry of Health and Housing until 1964. The change of name signifies the growth of the two departments.

8. It is not possible to deal here with the variety of interpretations which have been given to the term and meaning of African Socialism. The general principles of socialism were described as ownership and operation of fundamental means of production by the state, control of means of production, planning the use of resources in the interest of the people, distribution of income to avoid excessive concentration in the hands of a few, encouragement of cooperatives, and guarantees of equal opportunity without discrimination, KANU (Kenya African National Union) and the government were pledged to promote social advance by political means and by adherence to the African principle of individual service on behalf of the entirẽ community which would include community-based self-help or *Harambee.*

9. Tom Mboya, *The Challenge of Nationhood,* Praeger, New York, 1970, p. 87.

10. Republic of Kenya, Ministry of Health and Housing, *Annual Report,* 1963, p. 5.

11. Ibid., *Annual Report,* 1964, p. 1.

12. Tom Mboya, op. cit., p. 80.

13. For detail, see Republic of Kenya, Ministry of Health, *Health Services in Kenya,* 1971, pp. 1-5.

14. Ibid., Table 1, Population Distribution by Province; Table 4, Distribution of Rural Health Centers by Province; and Table 5, Estimated Central Government Expenditure on Health, Kenya 1969-1970.

15. Republic of Kenya, Ministry of Health, *Proposal for the Improvement of Rural Health Services and the Development of Rural Health Training Centres in Kenya, 1972.* The table of contents alone shows the departure from previous reports. It lists: Section 1: Introduction; section 2: Situation analysis; section 3: Systems design; section 4: Project structure; section 5: Financial implications.

16. Ibid., pp. 14, 24.

17. Ibid., p. 5.

18. Republic of Kenya, Ministry of Health, *Appendices to a Proposal for the Improvement of Rural Health Services and the Development of Rural Health Training Centres in Kenya,* Nairobi, 1st April 1973, 15, A, 3.

19. Ibid., B, 15, 17.

20. Ibid., B, 24.

21. WHO, *Primary Health Care,* A Joint Report by the Director-General of the World Health Organization and the Executive Director of the United Nations Children's Fund, 8, 9. Geneva, 1978. See also below pp. 56, 57.

22. Medical Training Centre, Nairobi, "Annual Graduation Day," November 1978, 105, mimeograph, Ministry of Health, Nairobi, 1978.

23. Republic of Kenya, *Development Plan, 1974-1978* (1974).

24. Ibid., part I, V.

25. Ibid., part II, p. 449.

26. Ibid., p. 452.

27. Ibid., Tables 20.2 and 20.3, Government Health Facilities and Central Government Health Staff.

28. Ibid., p. 461. This quote came from the section on health education which was taken very seriously. In order to reach 95 percent of the population, the entire health staff, including paramedical trainees, field and clinical health personnel and the department of education were to be enlisted in the information program.

29. *The Standard,* Nairobi, December 17, 1976. Joram Amadi, "This hospital is a disgrace." The *Standard* is the leading English language newspaper in Kenya.

30. *Institute of Development Studies,* Nairobi. Mbere, Special Rural Development Program, Review-Replan, 1973/74-1975/76. Typescipt.

31. WHO-UNICEF, Geneva, *Alma Ata. Primary Health Care,* Report of the International Conference on Primary Health Care, Alma-Ata, USSR, 6-12 September 1978.

32. Ibid., pp. 2, 3.

33. Ibid., p. 4.

34. Ibid., p. 5.

35. F. M. Mburu examined the gap between rhetoric and implementation in health development projects in a recent article "Rhetoric-Implementation Gap in Health Delivery for a Rural Population in a Developing Country," *Social Science and Medicine,* 15 A, 1979. He compared the valuable goals set forth for development planning with the statistics of achievements. He concluded that the disparity between urban and rural health resources and services could only be overcome if planners and administrators were willing to take political risks. Decisions involving the spending of funds in areas where they were most needed but where political influence was lacking implied a risk for government officials.
Ibid., p. 582.

CHAPTER 8: TRADITIONAL MEDICINE IN EAST AFRICA TODAY

1. Lloyd W. Swantz, "The Role of Medicine Man Among the Zaramo of Dar es Salaam," thesis, typescript, University of Dar es Salaam, 1974, p. 361.

2. E. N. Mshiu, "Traditional Medicine and Modern Medicine," typescript, Traditional Medicine Research Unit, 1978 and P. A. Kitundu, M.D., "Bagamoyo Kisarawe Survey of Traditional Medicine," 1978, Dar es Salaam.

3. See, for instance, Livingstone's drive to open up the Zambezi river area through commerce between 1849 and 1851 to save human lives. Or, reports by the Church Missionary Society in Kikuyu in the 1890s. And Rochus Schmidt on his experience in German East Africa, quoted in Ann Beck, *Medicine and Society in Tanganyika, 1890-1930,* American Philosophical Society, 1977, p. 10.

4. For an early example, take the Maji Maji Revolt in German East Africa, 1905/06. In this case, the magic factor considered dangerous was the occult power to protect men in their attack on German soldiers who were to be driven into the sea. See John Iliffe, *Tanganyika Under German Rule,* 1905-1912.

5. Kenya National Archives, DC/KBU 3/27. Political Recordbook, 1912, pp. 122-123.

6. On the circumcision controversy, see Ann Beck, "Some Observations on Jomo Kenyatta in Britain, 1929-1930," *Cahiers d'Etudes Africaines,* 22, 1966, Paris.

7. *Tanzania National Archives* (TNA), 16/5/7, p. 285, 1933.

8. Ibid., vol. II, pp. 210-214, 224-225, May-September 1933. The men were described as real crooks. They selected their victims under a cloud of secrecy and accused them of having medicine in their home. Since every African had some medicine in his home against unforeseen disasters, they collected fines from everyone present.

9. For the use of the term science, see below, p. 64.

10. Provincial Secretary Kitching, TNA 5/7/284, pp. 2, 3.

11. See, for instance, the articles which appeared in *Tanganyika Notes and Records* for 1930-1960; the *East African Medical Journal* for the same period; books by George W. Harley, *Native African Medicine,* E. E. Evans-Pritchard, *Witchcraft, Oracles, and Magic Among the Azande,* and Erwin Ackerknecht, *Medicine and Ethnology.* For detailed list, see bibliography.

12. Ackerknecht, *Medicine and Ethnology,* Johns Hopkins University Press, 1972, p. 135.

13. Ibid., p. 122.

14. TNA 21845, Folder Witchcraft, 12 October 1933.

15. Ibid. He may have emphasized herbal healing because the medical department was primarily interested in its role in traditional medicine, but he also may have thought that the magical character of traditional medicine would not be understood by the scientifically oriented doctor.

16. John S, Mbiti, *African Religions and Philosophy,* Heinemann, London, 1969.

17. Ibid., 75 ff.

18. Kitching in 1937. He reflected the ideas of Europeans. See above note 10.

19. Mbiti, op. cit., p. 84.

20. Swantz, Role of Medicine Man, pp. 178 ff.

21. C. K. Omari, "The Mganga: A Specialist of his own kind," *Psychopathologie Africaine,* 1972, VIII, 221.

22. Ibid., p. 220.

23. Evans-Pritchard, op. cit., p. 195.

24. P. J. Madati, "The Impact of Traditional Medicine on Managerial and Legal Aspects of Health Care Service in the Region," lecture, typescript, Central Government Chemical Laboratory, Dar es Salaam, 1978.

25. World Health Organizastion, "African Traditional Medicine," Technical Report Series, no. 1, p. 2.

26. Ibid., p. 1.

27. See TNA 21845, vol. I, 12 October 1933, "African Medicine," *Tanganyika Notes and Records,* various issues between 1936 and 1960. *East African Medical Journal,* Tanganyika Secretariat, Memoranda 1930-1955. East African Institute of Social Research, Sociology Papers 1959. Only literature of the British period is

cited here to indicate the status of traditional medicine as seen by contemporaries. Literature since 1961 will be cited below.

28. TNA, 13402/89, pp. 12-14.

29. See below on psychological value of supernatural treatment.

30. L. F. Gerlach, "Attitudes to Health and Disease among some East African Tribes," 1959, locus cited Makerere College. See also Erwin Ackerknecht, "The Rational in Primitive and the Supernatural in modern medicine," *Medicine and Ethnology,* pp. 160, 161 (1972).

31. "African Medicines," loc. cit., pp. 146-148.

32. Swantz, Role of Medicine Man, pp. 201, 202.

33. *Kenya and East African Medical Journal,* VII, 8, 1930, pp. 215-218.

34. TNA, 13402/89.

35. Dr. Weck, "Der Wahehe-Arzt in der Kaiserlichen Schutztruppe fur Deutsch-Ostafrika," *Deutsches Kolonialblatt,* 1908, pp. 1048-1051.

36. *Tanganyika Notes and Records*, W. D. Raymond, "Native Materia Medica," I, 1936, 1, pp. 77-80; II, TNR 1036 and III, 1938.

37. E. M. Mshiu, "Traditional Medicine and Modern Medicine," typescript, Dar es Salaam, p. 2, 1978.

38. TNA 21845, vol. I, November 1933.

39. Ibid., vol. II, November 1933.

40. See chapter 6, above pp. 80-81.

41. C. K. Omari, op. cit., 217.

42. *Tanganyika Notes and Records,* no. 66, 1966, pp. 193-201.

43. Ibid., 193.

44. See above chapter 8, section I.

45. Dr. K. Ndeti, "The Relevance of the African Traditional Doctor in Scientific Medicine," *African Sociology Papers,* Makerere Institute of Social Research, 1968/69, 378-390.

46. Ibid., p. 389.

47. Ibid., 390.

48. ARGUS, Uganda, July 14, 1964.

49. Mark T. Bura, a third-year medical student at the University of Dar es Salaam, "The Wairaqu Concepts of Causation, Diagnosis and Treatment of Disease," *Dar es Salaam Medical Journal,* vol. 6, 1, 1974.

50. Ibid., pp. 56-58.

51. J. G. A. J. Hautvast and L. J. Hautvast, "Analysis of a Bantu Medical System," A Nyakusa Case-Study (Tanzania), *Tropical and Geographical Medicine,* 1972, pp. 406-414.

52. The session with its blunt questions and answers is interesting in itself but cannot be presented in detail here.

53. Ibid., 413.

54. Cranford Pratt, *The Critical Phase in Tanzania, 1945-1968,* Cambridge University Press, 1976, ch. 8, "The commitment to socialism."

55. Arusha Declaration, Julius K. Nyerere, part one, *UJAMAA, Essays on Socialism,* Oxford University Press, 1968.

56. Dean McHenry, Jr., "The Struggle for Rural Socialism in Tanzania," pp. 31-61, *Socialism in Sub-Saharan Africa,* Carl Rosberg and Thomas Callaghy, ed., Institute of International Studies, UCLA, 1979.

57. See statements in the following: *African Traditional Medicine,* Afro Technical Report Series, no. 1. WHO, Brazzaville, 1976; Extract from WHO/AFRO Regional Committee meeting, Kampala, Uganda, September, 1976; E. N. Mshiu, Director, Traditional Medicine Research Unit, University of Dar es Salaam, "Traditional Medicine and Modern Medicine," typescript, 1978; P. S. Madati, "The Impact of Traditional Medicine on Management and Legal Aspects of Health Care Services in the Region," Dar es Salaam, 1978.

58. Madati, op. cit., appendix 1 and 2.

59. Mshiu, op. cit., p. 3.

60. Z. A. Ademuwagun, "The Challenge of the Existence of Orthodox and Traditional Medicine in Nigeria," *The African Medical Journal,* 1976, p. 21.

61. Swantz, Role of Medicine Man, p. 144.

62. Ibid., 338-339.

63. E. N. Mshiu listed among the objections by doctors their fear that association with traditional healers would undermine the accepted value system of scientific medicine. Also apprehension that tolerance of traditional practices whose outcome had not been scientifically demonstrated would make the cooperating doctor guilty of human experimentation. And finally, the danger that traditional practices might be contrary to standards which the modern doctor was legally and ethically bound to observe.

64. Minister of Health A. H. Mwinyi cited targets of 16,000 health and health-related personnel to be trained between 1973 and 1980 while F. D. E. Mtango quoted as targets for 1980 a total of 700 doctors, 1,200 medical assistants, 2,800 rural medical aides, 600 nurses, 200 health officers and health auxiliaries, altogether 6,000 people. See Speech by Minister of Health, Hon. A. H. Mwinyi for the Financial Year 1974/75, p. 40. Government Publication, Dar es Salaam, 1973; and F. D. Mtango, "The Role of the Doctor in Rural Health Services: Providing Scientific Medicine through Medical Auxiliaries," p. 1. Unpublished manuscript, Dar es Salaam.

65. Bagamoyo Field Project, "A Study of Common Medical Conditions Attended by Traditional Healers in Kerege and Zinga Villages in September 1979." Unpublished Seminar Project, University of Dar es Salaam.

CHAPTER 9: CONCLUSIONS

1. See, for instance, Malcolm Segall, "The Politics of Health in Tanzania," in *Towards Socialist Planning,* ed. by J. F. Rweyemamu and others, 1974, Tanzania Publishing House.

2. Dean E. McHenry, Jr., "The Struggle for Rural Socialism in Tanzania," in Carl Rosberg and Thomas M. Callaghy, ed., *Socialism in Subsaharan Africa,* University of California, 1979.

3. Ibid., pp. 43 and 60. After a slow start, peasant movement to Ujamaas reached 47.5 percent between mid-1974 and mid-1975, then declined to 24. percent between mid-1975 and mid-1976, and reached a high of 91.3 percent in 1977.

4. Ibid., p. 60.

5. *Daily News,* Dar es Salaam, article by Isaac Mruma, December 1977.

6. See above , chapter 6.

7. See Republic of Kenya, *Ministry of Health, Health Services in Kenya,* 1971 and idem, *Proposal for the Improvement of Health Services and the Development of Rural Health Training Centers in Kenya,* 1972; idem, *Appendices to a Proposal for the Improvement of Rural Health Services and the Development of Rural Health Training Centres in Kenya,* 1973.

8. During a visit to Nairobi in 1979, I had an opportunity to observe meetings conducted by Dr. Kanani, Deputy Director for Health. Most impressive is the method by which technical leadership is exercised by community-selected trainees on all levels. Small units outside the capital were made aware of their potential for effective input by carrying out health auxiliary activities and communicating directly with the responsible officials in Nairobi. Equally significant has been the work of the Medical Training Center that operates in the opposite direction, from the center to the periphery.

9. See chapter 7, above.

10. Ann Beck, *A History of the British Medical Administration in East Africa,* 1900-1970, Harvard University Press, 1970, pp. 76-81.

11. One has only to think of the East African Medical Research Council under the East African Community.

12. They were: The East African Virus Research Institute at Entebbe in Uganda; The East African Trypanosomiasis Research Organization at Tororo in Uganda; The East African Tuberculosis Investigation Centre in Nairobi, Kenya; the East African Leprosy Research Centre at Alupe in Kenya; The East African Institute of Malaria and Vector Borne Diseases in Amani, Tanzania; and The Tropical Pesticides Research Institute in Arusha. See James M. Gekonyo, "Organization and Management of Medical Research in Kenya," paper presented at First Annual Medical Scientific Conference of Kenya Medical Research Institute and Kenya Trypanosomiasis Research Institute, 1980, p. 6.

13. Ibid., p. 13. See also F. Kamunvi, "Some Organizational and Operational Constraints in the Former Regional Research Organization." First Annual Medical Scientific Conference, Nairobi, 1980.

14. A. N. Nhonoli, "Medical and Technological Research in Relation to Regional Cooperation and Primary Health," First Annual Medical Scientific Conference, Nairobi, 1980, Chairman's Address, p. 6.

15. Ibid., p. 12.

16. Ministry of Health, Dar es Salaam, Speech by Minister of Health Ndugu Leader Stirling, M.P. for the financial year 1976/77, pp. 31 and 43.

17. Deputy Director S. Kanani, "Primary Health Care, the Kenya Experience," International Conference on Primary Health Care, Alma Ata, USSR, September 1978. (Ministry of Health, Kenya).

REFERENCES

GOVERNMENT DOCUMENTS.

Unpublished sources and Official Publications for Kenya, Tanganyika and East Africa, 1920-1960.

Historical Documents

Indians in Kenya. Memorandum on Native Policy in East Africa. Cmd. 1922. 1923.

Report of the East Africa Commission. Cmd. 2387. 1925.

Future Policy in Regard to Eastern Africa. Cmd. 2904. 1927.

Native Affairs Department. Annual Report for East Africa, 1927.

Report of the Commission on Closer Union of the Dependencies in Eastern and Central Africa, 1928-1929. Cmd. 3234. 1929. (Also cited as Hilton Young Report.)

Report of Sir Samuel Wilson on his Visit to East Africa, 1929. Cmd. 3378.

Memorandum on Native Policy in East Africa. Cmd. 3573. 1930.

Report by Joint Select Committee on Closer Union in East Africa, 1931. House of Lords 184.

Certain Questions in Kenya. Report by Financial Commissioner Lord Moyne. Cmd. 4093, 1931.

The Colonial Empire. Cmd. 7167. 1946-1947.

Reports Relating to Development

Colonial Development Advisory Committee, First Interim Report 1929-1930. Cmd. 3540.

Third Interim Report 1931-1932. Cmd. 4079.

Statement of Policy on Colonial Development and Welfare. Cmd. 6175. 1939-1940.

Eleventh and Final Report for 1939-1940. Cmd. 6298. 1941.

Colonial Development and Welfare Act, 1940: Return of Schemes for period 1945-1946. Cmd. 1946.

Colonial Development and Welfare, Despatch by Secretary of State for the Colonies to Colonial Governments. Cmd. 6713. 1945.

Colony and Protectorate of Kenya, Development and Reconstruction Authority Report, 1947 (1948).

GOVERNMENT PUBLICATIONS BY KENYA (COLONY AND PROTECTORATE), 1920-1963.

The *Annual Medical Reports* were published by the Colonial Medical Department up to 1962. Thereafter they were published by the Medical Department of the Republic of Kenya. Reports cited or used in part are listed below:

Annual Medical Reports for 1926, 1928, 1933-1937, 1953, 1962, 1964 and Ministry of Health, *Health Services in Kenya*–1971.

Ministry of Health, *Proposal for the Improvement of the Rural Health Services and the Development of Rural Training Centres in Kenya, 1972.*

Ministry of Health, *Appendices to A Proposal for the Improvement of Rural Health Training Centres in Kenya,* 1973.

Republic of Kenya, *Development Plan for the Period 1974-1978,* Nairobi, 1978.

UNPUBLISHED MATERIAL IN THE TANZANIA NATIONAL ARCHIVES, DAR ES SALAAM.

Tanzania National Archives, Folder on Witchcraft. File 16/5/7, Correspondence between Provincial Commissioner and District Officers, 1933-1944.

TNA, 13350. Rural Health Services, 1951.

TNA, 26854. Central Development Committee, 1939.

TNA, 12602. Correspondence Sneath with Provincial Office, 1946-1951.

TNA, 13571. Correspondence on Native Administration, Tribal Dressers, Rural Medical Services, 1928-1955.

SECONDARY SOURCES.

Ackernecht, Erwin H. *Medicine and Ethnology.* Selected Essays. Baltimore: The Johns Hopkins Press, 1971.

Ademuwagun, Z. A. "The Challenge of the Coexistence of Orthodox and Traditional Medicine in Nigeria." *The East African Medical Journal* (1976): 21-32.

Amery, L. S. *My Political Life.* vol. 2. London: Hutchinson, 1953.

Beck, Ann. *A History of the British Medical Administration, 1900-1950.* Cambridge: Harvard University Press, 1970.

_____. *Medicine and Society in Tanganyika, 1890-1930.* Philadelphia: The American Philosophical Society, 1977.

_____. "History of Medicine and Health Services in Kenya, 1900-1950." *In Health and Disease in Kenya.* Nairobi: East African Literature Bureau, 1974.

Black, Cyril E. *The Dynamics of Modernization.* Princeton: Princeton University Press, 1967.

Brett, E. A. *Colonialism and Underdevelopment in East Africa: The Politics of Economic Change.* 1919-1939. New York: NOK Publishers, 1973.

Cell, John W., ed. *By Kenya Possessed: The Correspondence of Norman Leys and J. H. Oldham,* 1918-1926. Chicago: The University of Chicago Press, 1976.

Cliffe, Lionel et al., eds. *Rural Cooperation in Tanzania.* Dar es Salaam: Tanzania Publishing House, 1975.

Cliffe, Lionel and John S. Saul, eds. *Socialism in Tanzania,* vols. 1 and 2. Dar es Salaam; East African Publishing House, 1972, 1973.

Cohen, Sir Andrew. *British Policy in Changing Africa.* London: Routledge and Kegan Paul, 1959.

East African Council for Medical Research. Annual Reports for 1955-1960. Nairobi.

East African High Commission 1961-1976. Arusha: East African Common Service.

East African Medical Journal: Nairobi, Kenya. vol. 1940-1960.

Ellman, A. O. "Progress and Prospects in Ujamaa Development in Tanzania." In Lionel Cliffe et al., eds., *Rural Cooperation in Tanzania,* Dar es Salaam: Tanzania Publishing House, 1975.

Van Etten, G. M. *Rural Health Development in Tanzania.* Amsterdam: Van Gorcum. 1976.

Gekonyo, James S. "Organization and Management of Medical Research in Kenya." Paper read at First Annual Medical Scientific Conference. Nairobi, 1980. (unpublished)

Gerlach, L. F. "Attitudes to Health and Disease among Some East African Tribes." *Sociology Papers,* 1959. Kampala: East African Institute of Social Research.

Gish, Oscar. *Planning the Health Sector, The Tanzanian Experience.* Croom Helm Ltd., 1975, 1978.

Goulet, Denis. *The Cruel Choice: A New Concept in the Theory of Development.* New York: Atheneum, 1975.

Gutkind, Peter and Immanuel Wallerstein, eds. *The Political Economy of Contemporary Africa.* Beverly Hills: Sage Publications, 1976.

Hailey, W. M. *An African Survey.* London: Oxford University Press, 1956.

Harley, George W. *Native African Medicine.* London: Frank Cass and Co. 1970.

Hautvast, J. G. A. and L. J. Hautvast. "Analysis of a Bantu Medical System." London: *Tropical and Geographical Medicine.* 1972.

Iliffe, John. *Tanganyika under German Rule. 1905-1912.* Cambridge: Cambridge University Press, 1969.

Institute of Development Studies, Mbera, "Special Rural Development Programme Review-Replan. 1973/74-1975/76." Typescript. Nairobi.

Imperato, P. J. "Witchcraft and Traditional Medicine among the Luo of Tanzania." Dar es Salaam: Tanzania Notes and Records, 66, 1966.

Jansen, G. *The Doctor-Patient Relationship in an African Tribal Society.* Assen: Van Gorcum, 1973.

Kamunvi, Fabian. "Main Landmarks in the Development of Medical Research in East Africa." Nairobi: 1st Annual Medical Scientific Conference. Nairobi, 1980.

———. "Some of the Important Contributions of Medical Research in East Africa." Nairobi: 1st Annual Medical Scientific Conference. Nairobi, 1980.

Kanani, S. "Primary Health Care, The Kenya Experience"; Ministary of Health, Nairobi, 1978.

Kaplinski, R. M. "Ideology in Development Theory." Nairobi: Institute for Development Studies, Working Paper no. 224. 1975.

Kjekshus, Helge. *Ecology Control and Economic Development in East African History. The Case of Tanganyika, 1850-1950.* Berkeley: University of California Press, 1977.

Latham, Michael C. "Priorities for Nutrition and Health Programmes in Africa." Boston: African Studies Association Paper, 1976.

Lee, J. M. *Colonial Development and Good Government: A Study of Ideas Expressed by the British Official Classes in Planning Decolonization, 1939-1964.* Oxford University Press, 1967.

Legislative Council of Tanganyika. "A Review of the Medical Policy of Tanganyika." 1949: Government Printer. Dar es Salaam.

Leys, Colin. "The Political Climate for Economic Development," *African Affairs,* 1966.

——. *Underdevelopment in Kenya. The Political Economy of Neo-Colonialism.* Berkeley: University of California Press, 1975.

McHenry, Dean E., Jr. *Tanzania's Ujamaa Villages.* Berkeley: University of California Press. 1979.

——. "The Struggle for Rural Socialism in Tanzania" in *Socialism in Sub-Saharan Africa.* Berkeley: University of California Press, 1979.

McLean, Una. *Magical Medicine. A Nigerian Case Study.* Alan Lane: The Penguin Press, 1971.

Mascarenhas, Ophelia. *A Preliminary Guide to the Study of Traditional Medicine in Tanzania.* Dar es Salaam: Bureau of Resource Assessment and Land Use Planning, 1975.

Mboya, Tom. *The Challenge of Nationhood.* New York: Praeger Publishers, 1970.

Mbiti, John S. *African Religions and Philosophy.* London: Heinemann, 1969.

Mburu, F. M. "Rhetoric Implementation Gap in Health Policy and Health Services Delivery for a Rural Population," First Annual Medical Scientific Conference. Nairobi, 1980.

Middleton, John. *The Effects of Economic Development on Traditional Political Systems in Africa South of the Sahara.* London: Mouton, 1966.

Middleton, John and E. H. Winter. *Witchcraft and Sorcery in East Africa.* London: Routledge & Keegan Paul. 1963.

Moore, Sally Faulk and Paul Puritt. *The Chagga and Meru of Tanzania.* London: International Institute. 1977.

Mshiu, E. N. "Traditional Medicine and Modern Medicine." (typescript) University of Dar es Salaam. 1978.

Mtango, F. D. "The Role of the Doctor in Rural Health Services: Scientific Medicine through Medical Auxiliaries," unpulished paper. University of Dar es Salaam. 1978.

Mwinyi, Hon. A. H Budget Speech by the Minister for Health for the Year 1972/73. Dar es Salaam, 1972. Government of Tanzania.

——. Budget Speech by the Minister of Health, for the Year 1973/74, Dar es Salaam, 1973.

——. Budget Speech by the Minister for Health for the Year 1974/75, Dar es Salaam, 1974.

Navarro, Vincente. "The Underdevelopment of Health: An Analysis of the Distribution of Health Resources in Latin America." International Journal of Health Services, 1974: Farmingdale, N Y.

Ndeti, K. "The Relevance of the African Traditional Doctor in Scientific Medicine." *African Sociology Papers,* 1968/69: Makerere Institute of Social Research.

Nhonoli, A. M. "Medical and Technological Research in Relation to Regional Cooperation and Primary Health." 1980: First Annual Scientific Conference. Nairobi.

Nyerere, Julius K. *Ujamaa–Essays on Socialism.* London: Oxford University Press, 1968.

———. *Man and Development.* London: Oxford University Press, 1974.

Omari, C. K. "The Mwanga: A Specialist of His Own Kind." *Psychopathologie Africaine,* Dar es Salaam. 1972.

Pratt, Cranford. *The Critical Phase in Tanzania 1945-1968: Nyerere and the Emergence of a Socialist Strategy.* Cambridge: Cambridge University Press, 1976.

Rweyemamu, Justinian. *Underdevelopment and Industrialization in Tanzania.* London: Oxford University Press, 1973.

Schulpen, T. W. J. *Integration of Church and Government Medical Services.* Nairobi: African Medical Research Foundation, 1975.

Smith, Hadley E. *Readings of Economic Development and Administration in Tanzania.* Dar es Salaam, 1966.

Sorokin, Alan L. *Health Economics in Developing Countries.* Lexington: Lexington Books, 1977.

Stirling, Leader, M.P. Budget Speech by the Minister for Health, for the Financial Year 1976/1977: Government of Tanzania, Dar es Salaam.

Streeten, Paul. "Changing Perceptions of Development." *Finance and Development.* 14:14-16, 1977.

Swantz, Lloyd W. *The Role of Medicine Man Among the Zaramo of Dar es Salaam.* Unpublished Ph.D. thesis, 1974: University of Dar es Salaam.

Swynnerton, R. J. N. "A Plan to Intensify the Development of African Agriculture in Kenya." Nairobi: Government Printer, 1955.

Tanzania Notes and Records. The Journal of the Tanzania Society. Dar es Salaam.

Titmuss, Richard. *The Health Services of Tanganyika.* London: Pitman Medical Publishing Co., 1964.

Weck. "Der Wahehe Arzt in der Kaiserlichen Schutztuppe fur Deutsch-Ostafrika." Berlin: Deutsches Kolonialblatt. 1908.

World Health Organization. *African Traditional Medicine.* Brazzaville: Afro-Technical Report Series, no. 1, 1976.

———. *Primary Health Care. Report of the International Conference at Alma Ata (USSR).* 1978: WHO Geneva, 1978.

———. *Primary Health Care. Joint Report by the Director General of WHO and the Executive Director of UNICEF.* Geneva: WHO, 1978.

———. *Tropical Diseases Today.* Geneva: WHO. 1975.

INDEX

ABOUT THE AUTHOR

Ann Beck, Professor of History Emeritus at the University of Hartford, has taught British colonial history and African history since 1950. She has devoted the last fifteen years entirely to research on East Africa and the role of medicine in its history. During her research, she visited Kenya and Tanzania extensively on twelve occasions. Dr. Beck received her graduate degrees from the University of Illinois (Phi Beta Kappa). She is a member of the African Studies Association, the American Association for the History of Medicine, and a co-founder of the Connecticut Valley African Colloquium. She is the author of *A History of the British Medical Administration of East Africa, 1908-1950*; *Medicine and Society in Tanganyika, 1890-1930*; and a contributor to *Health and Disease in Kenya*, published in Nairobi. She also has published numerous articles on Africa.